Momentum: A Model for Motivation in Rehabilitation

for Individuals with Traumatic Brain Injury

by

Lynda Gail Cleveland, B.A., M.A.

Dissertation

Presented to the Faculty of the Graduate School of

The University of Texas at Austin

in Partial Fulfillment

of the Requirements

for the Degree of

Doctor of Philosophy

The University of Texas at Austin

May, 1998

Momentum: A Model for Motivation in Rehabilitation for Individuals with Traumatic Brain Injury

Lynda G. Cleveland, PhD

Detour Ahead Press
Austin, Texas
sales@detourpress.org
www.detourpress.org

ISBN: 0-9777795-9-9

Detour Ahead Press Edition

Original Cover Graphic
M. Kevin Ford

Production & Publishing Services
Groundbreaking Press
www.groundbreaking.com

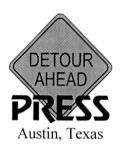

Austin, Texas

Momentum: A Model for Motivation in Rehabilitation for Individuals with Traumatic Brain Injury

Approved by
Dissertation Committee:

Diane Lemonnier Schallert, Supervisor

Frank W. Wicker

Mary F. Whiteside

Judith B. Harris

Dedication

In memory of

my grandparents

Dr. and Mrs. C. M. Cleveland

and

my dad

Ray O. Cleveland

In honor of

my folks

Mr. and Mrs. Henry D. Rutledge

Acknowledgements

"Bless the Lord, O my soul: and all that is within me bless His Holy name. Bless the Lord, O my soul, and forget not all His benefits: who forgiveth all thine iniquities; who healeth all thy diseases; Who redeemeth thy life from destruction; who crowneth thee with loving kindness and tender mercies; Who satisfieth thy mouth with good things; so that thy youth is renewed like the eagle's."

from a psalm of David (103:1-5)

How could I fail to give God glory and praise

He has truly saved my soul by the gift of love through Jesus,

And indeed healed me from great tragedy.

Yes, He has redeemed me from destruction

And I shall praise the Lord through my entire sojourn on this earth!

How could I not show gratitude and adoration to Him

    for all the benefits of His love to me?

from a psalm of Lynda

In the New Testament, Jesus gave us the story of the Good Samaritan. As Jesus told the story there was a man going down from Jerusalem to Jericho and he fell among thieves who robbed him and took all his possessions; they beat him and left him for dead. A priest passed by on one side and a Levite passed by on the other side and neither bothered to pause. But a certain Samaritan came along and had compassion on the one who had been left for dead. He bound up his wounds, poured in oil and wine, picked him up, sat him on his own beast, and brought him to an inn and took care of him. When the Samaritan had to leave, he gave the Innkeeper two pence and said to him, "take care of him and when I return, if he owes you more, I will pay you."

How are those who ponder this story able to understand the perspective of the one who received such mercy unless they have been likewise assisted?

Many times since 1984 I have felt like the one who was robbed, beaten, and left near death. The acknowledgements for this dissertation would be tragically incomplete if I did not share a glimpse from among the vast number and diversity of ministering souls God provided since that bleak day in 1984.

In Chapter 1, I recount my involvement in a near fatal motor vehicle accident in 1984 in Melbourne, Australia. I was pulled from the wreck not expected to live, but the paramedics did a marvelous job in transporting me to the Dandenong and District Hospital where I received the finest in emergency medical care. As I began my rehabilitation journey I did not know it would span more than a decade, or that strategically deployed Good Samaritans would be posted by God at exact intervals to attend to me. These Good Samaritans have assisted me in achieving this doctoral goal. One I set in a hospital bed in 1984.

Almost from the moment of impact, a host of gifted physicians and rehabilitation specialists have assisted me. From among them, I offer special thanks to Dr. Eng-Seong Tan of St. Vincent's Hospital and Miss F. Nora Ley, R.N., formerly of Epworth Hospital, both of Melbourne, Australia. Treatment for traumatic brain injury was not as advanced at the time of my accident as it is now; however, these two were perceptive in their diagnosis of the severe brain injury amidst the multitude of physical injuries I had sustained, and tenacious in their treatment. Over the years Nora, in particular, became far more than my nurse: she became my friend. I shall always be indebted to her.

To be injured thousands of miles away from your homeland is traumatic enough, but to be hospitalized in a foreign land without your family makes it worse. God, in His infinite wisdom, sent throngs of Good Samaritans my way. Fellow church members in Syndal Baptist Church, Melbourne never left me to wonder if I was loved or cared for. My intent is to offer my heartfelt thanks to all of that congregation who gave of themselves by naming representatives: the pastoral staff and several with whom I've stayed in touch over the years: the late Rev. Robert McMillan, Rev. Dr. Geoff Blackburn, Rev. Dr. Bill Brown, Warren Smith and family, Dawn, Grant and Fiona Burrows, and Heather and Carl Bray.

Eight years after my injury, I was finally discharged by my Australian physicians. The fellowship of my home church, First Baptist Church, Dallas, blanketed me with love and reassurances that I could overcome the injuries and tragedies of 1984. Friends, like Kay Dosterschill and her family, who had known me before were supportive in my attempts to resume a "normal" lifestyle. I was not allowed to drive, Good Samaritans transported me. I fought to remember simple things we take for granted each day, Good Samaritans retaught me. Each step of the way, God provided encouragers. Often, a card would arrive in the mail from members of my Mother's Sunday school class; (what a wealth of "mothers" they've been to me!) God knew when the Good Samaritan touch of comfort was needed. My awed thanks to Carolyn Selzer for her attentiveness over the years, for her discernment in knowing when those cards were needed. She orchestrated the first cards the very week I was injured in 1984; I received the most recent one last week: the morning I defended this dissertation. God is so good!

The marvelous and indefinable uniqueness of God's all sufficient grace is illustrated by the variety of Good Samaritans He has stationed to attend me worldwide. For me, His support system has extended from Australia to Dallas to Austin. I had been advised time and again I'd never regain my independence, but thanks to the efforts of Dr. Hal Unwin and Dr. Lawrence Brazune, seizures have been brought under control and I have regained an exciting life. These fine physicians always encouraged me, and were always there when I needed medical assistance. Maureen Gordon, formerly Dr. Barzune's assistant, not only was attentive medically, but was a special booster in helping me regain my public speaking skills. My first venture back into the "work world" was afforded through the watchcare of the volunteer division, under the direction of Catherine Bywaters at Presbyterian Hospital, Dallas. The staff there, especially in the Emergency Department where I worked, gently retaught me many skills, while allowing me to feel important. I thank them.

When I moved to Austin, my lifelong friends, Barbara and Jim Word, provided me the privilege of room and board in their home. Thanks to Barb's patience and teaching I reconstructed much of my past and continued to strengthen the foundation for regaining independence. Thank you Barb and Jim for the hours you spent in rebuilding and encouraging.

At First Baptist Church, Austin, friends who had known my grandparents welcomed me weekly at church and knew just when I needed a boost. Two very special Good Samaritans, Frances and Mildred Jackson, "adopted me" and strengthened me during my sojourn through graduate school. They have been my family here; I know I can call on them anytime for anything.

The support network God unfolded had many faces and occupations. Consider the trio at the local Texaco: Stacy, Mark, and the manager, Darrell Coe: they've lent real fuel to my doctoral journey - like keeping Old Blue running until the Black Beauty appeared, which brings me to yet another set of God's suppliers: the folks at Mercedes Benz Corporation. A special thanks to Barry Layton (Australia), and to Jeff Cunningham (Austin, USA) for their willingness to be used in God's supply line, in His design for my doctoral aspirations. God knew a dependable car was critical to data gathering!

Good Samaritans from every walk of life were on each corner cheering me on in pursuit of this doctoral dream. Confinement in a body and neck brace often makes one feel less than beautiful; however, God provided tender care and esteem boosters through friends at Northlake Beauty Salon (Dallas) especially Rita, Lorane, Diana, Rosemary, Marie, Linda, Liz and Ruby. Martha Coleman, my Austin landlord, became a friend, was always available to lift my spirits, and sought to care for my dwelling so the dissertation rhythm was not disturbed. Wonderful were the friends who cared for Jessye, my medical service dog–an eight pound black poodle: Jessye's groomer, Florence "Mimi" Haefele, the friends at Brykerwood Veterinary Clinic (Austin), and Abrams Veterinary Clinic (Dallas). The folks at Southwest Airlines likewise have been accommodating of Jessye. They reap my appreciation and oodles of poodle praises, too.

Then there are my Media lab buddies: Glenda Garcia, Ingrid Martin, Mary Ann Forestell, Angie Jimenez-Espinoza, Norma Castillo Casas, Valerie Whiting, Natalie Villon, Mike Bell, Carlos Colon, Ken Waters and Elsa Alonso. A special thanks to Glenda who labored shoulder to shoulder with me at work as well as the research field keeping me organized and energized. For Glenda and the media staff, the camaraderie we enjoyed this year and the support they offered defy description.

Sometimes God sends a Good Samaritan with just an encouraging word. I learned the smile we offer others may be the very tool God uses. I received a motivational charge on a daily basis in the form of warm greetings from Nona, Myra, Sandy, Linda and Claire. That makes them encouragers in word as well as deed as these secretaries have helped me function within the system.

One truly dedicated friend and faithful Samaritan is Pattie Rose. Hers was the first voice of UT I heard; her attentiveness made a profound impression. Throughout my UT academic journey she carefully advised, guided, trained, cautioned, and cheered me on. And who do you suppose came through with the final touches on this document? Pattie arranged all the formatting, proofread multiple versions, consulted on and verified APA style sheet as well as graduate specifications... if the value of souls were to be calculated in hours spent in labor, Pattie Rose and Esther Yacono would be inestimable. Esther Yacono transcribed all the data and proofread the manuscript.

A very special independent tribute should be made to Esther without whose help this goal would not have been achieved this May. Esther spent untold hours transcribing 64 hours of audiotape. Her insights into the relationships were an added bonus as was her attentiveness and concern as I debriefed regularly from emotionally draining days in the field. Esther, this goal was attainable May, 1998 largely because of your efforts. Thank you.

Not only did God provide excellent help right here in Austin, but from UT Southwestern Medical Center in Dallas, Jeanne Moore served as an outside reader to survey my grounded theory audit trail. Jeanne, a neurorehabilitation specialist offered her knowledgeable touch not only to the manuscript, but also to assisting my personal physical navigation of this journey. Inspired editors are indeed a gift from God.

God's messengers surely included my graduate colleagues, especially Mike Harris and Barbara Holmes. Mike and I ran the academic obstacle course together assisting and cheering one another on. His sense of humor often lightened the load, especially in the home stretch. A special thanks to my friend and "dissertation cheerleader," Barbara Holmes, Ph.D., R.N., who allowed me to sit in on her final orals in 1996, and who has coached me every step of the way since then. God sends such Samaritans on trailblazing missions of mercy that only they can fulfill.

At the administrative level, God provided unexpected help, too, in Vice President and Graduate Dean Teresa Sullivan, and in the Doctoral Evaluator, Lynn Renegar. I thank each of them for their availability to meet special needs behind the scenes known only to Him.

I regret I cannot name one of the most significant groups of Good Samaritans because of the need to protect their privacy. However, to each participant in all three studies, I offer special thanks. You are the heart and soul of this dissertation and I will be eternally grateful to each of you for allowing me to enter into your lives, walk with you awhile, and learn from you. The staff of the facility where I gathered data treated me as one of their own and always made me feel welcome. The staff and residents all exhibited an enthusiasm for my research that was a source of extra energy. The Chief Executive Officer of the rehabilitation facility where I spent nine months was especially a Godsend. This gifted physician carefully shepherded me along the way in research, as well as overseeing my own professional growth in the field of neurorehabilitation. Because I cannot call him by name, I'll simply say, "Please know, Doc, that you hold a very special spot in the final stages of my own recovery and the initial stages of my work in neurorehabilitation. I will always be grateful."

I have cited only a representative portion of the globe-stretching network of supporters I've been blessed with at every stage of my recovery journey. Yet, none are greater Samaritans than the ones God gave me even before this life-changing crisis occurred. Outside of my salvation, the greatest gift God has given me is a Christian home. My brother, Kenneth, and I have been taught by our parents' example and nurtured in God's love throughout our lives. We were encouraged to be the very best we could be, and every opportunity for physical, spiritual and intellectual growth was afforded us. How many times did we hear,

"The sky's the limit!"? Through happy times and sad, we were taught that "all things work together for good to them that love God, to them who are called according to His purpose." (Romans 8:28) This was a difficult truth to understand in 1978 when our Dad died suddenly of an apparent heart attack at the age of 58 in the prime of life. Though we were adults, Ken and I looked to Mom for strength. Solomon describes the characteristics of a godly woman in Proverbs 31:10-31. He must have been thinking of my mom when He wrote it. Mom did not fail us. She was the strength and guide even in those darkest of days. In these years of my recovery, Mom has been not only a caregiver, but my encourager, my confidant, my seamstress, my cheerleader, my critic, my advisor, my taxi driver, my banker, my business manager, and my sounding board, to name a few of her varied talents. Mom has a unique way of saying, "I love you. Go for it," with a surprise note in the mail, a new blouse for no reason, a shared day shopping, or by preparing and freezing forty meals so I would not have to cook during my dissertation writing days. My mom and I are best friends. When I think of all the Good Samaritan "lifts" I've received, the memory I shall treasure most from my doctoral pursuit, is the day I walked into a room at my mom's house unexpectedly and heard her praying for me. What a precious gift; one I shall never forget.

In the years following my Dad's death, my mom remarried. A friend of over three decades through church activities, Henry D. Rutledge became my father, "by-law." I rejoiced that my mom was once again happy; but I never imagined God had prepared her husband to also be a most significant Good Samaritan in my future path. The union of his family and ours over these last sixteen years has been one of the most exciting of God's blessings: no longer two families, but one, complete with the older sister I never had. Henry, my "father", has been enthusiastic for all of my endeavors; he has been a willing editor on every paper in this doctoral pursuit; he has never let me think of giving up; he always been willing to listen, to brainstorm on projects; to reeducate me in areas my own TBI has left void. I do not think my own Dad could have been more supportive. I have been richly blessed.

To my brother Kenneth and his family, Terri, Danica and Colton, I thank you for always assuming I would some day achieve this goal, when I'm sure at times it looked uncertain. Ken, thanks for the example you set in daring to chase your dreams, it gave me strength.

To my older sister, Paula and her husband John, I thank you for your unquestioning support and for never asking, "are you ever going to get out of school?" Paula, for our "sister times," I am especially thankful.

And to my nephew and his wife, Todd and Angie, thank you for always bringing laughter into Aunt LuLu's life - you relieved a lot of tensions along the way.

Certainly acknowledgments would not be complete without a special tribute to those academicians who guided me on the right path. My doctoral pursuit had a positive, supportive beginning at the University of Texas Southwestern Graduate School of Biomedical Sciences, under the tutelage of Jim Battles, Ph.D., Anthony Frisbie, Ed.D., and Mary F. Whiteside, Ph.D.

The years I've spent on the Forty Acres I have been fortunate in "professorial" experiences. DeLayne Hudspeth carefully guided my program and encouraged my interdisciplinary aspirations. DeLayne, (TGWF), thank you for your support and willingness to help, no matter whether the request was to consult on Old Blue, or role play final orals. I gained valuable experience in structural decomposition and evaluation from Gary Borich. Ed Emmer orchestrated my growth in qualitative methods not only with his class, but also in his willingness to answer my questions all along the research journey. Anne Seraphine's bubbly free spirit and her enthusiasm for quantitative analysis were contagious. Elaine Fowler-Costas, C & I Graduate Adviser, guided me along the journey and supported my foray into the wilds of an interdisciplinary program.

Finally, I applaud my dissertation committee. Even my Synonym Finder cannot offer superlatives deserved by this group. I was blessed with a working committee. They tempered me; they tested me; they refined me; they polished me; they stretched me. I have had a delightful, though not trouble-free dissertation journey, and I thank each of you individually and corporately for prodding and steadying me all the way to the finish.

A special thanks to Mary Whiteside, Ph.D. When I first met Mary at UTSWMCD, I was unable to drive, and often had difficulty stringing sufficient thoughts together to carry on extended conversations. Mary patiently taught me many of the compensatory strategies I've employed throughout this rigorous journey. From teaching me to read at a graduate level, to encouraging me just moments before the oral defense of my dissertation, Mary was there for me, not only academically, but as a friend, a mentor who looked past the struggling TBI individual to the person with potential within. Thank you, Mary, for having confidence in me, often beyond my own estimation of my capacity. I was fortunate that God allowed you not only to direct my doctoral pursuit from the beginning, but also to serve on my dissertation committee. You did, in the Samaritan sense of the word, "pick me up" on the doctoral road and help me all along the way.

My enthusiasm for studying the reasons motivation worked, (hmmm, like a bellows to a fire), was fanned by Frank Wicker, Ph.D. Thank you, Frank, for your quick dry wit and synthesis questions that always kept me on my mental feet and made learning like an exciting scavenger hunt, always looking for the next treasure you would uncover. I gained valuable experience of analysis when you taught me "it depends."

It seems only fitting that God would also use the narrowing of my research topic to introduce me to another committee member, Sue Grobe, Ph.D. I was introduced to Sue by one of her colleagues in a distant city. She has proven to have a stabilizing influence on me personally as well as academically. She has been wise in pacing me. Her gentle redirection and insistence that I stay with the program have been important to the completion of my research. Thank you, Sue, for your sensitivity to the needs of individuals in rehabilitation, and for your patience in explanations.

Life has often been compared to a tapestry that we can only see from underneath, while God alone sees the beautiful weaving from above. I have a better appreciation for this analogy now because of the untimely tragic accident of Liu, Min, Ed.D. Liu, Min was a special spark on my committee; she's been instrumental since my early graduate days at Texas in rebuilding my self-confidence and self-esteem. Six weeks prior to my completion of this study, Liu, Min herself unexpectedly entered the world of which I had written - the realm of lengthy rehabilitation. While her injuries were to her spinal cord and not her brain, the heartache of disability was the same life-shattering trauma. Now, it was my turn to be a Good Samaritan to another in need, but try as I did, it was I, again, who received the blessings. Liu, Min's indomitable spirit and determination were and continue to be an inspiration to me. She remained on my committee, and her signature was the highlight of my defense day. For your courage, spirit, and determination, Liu, Min, I salute you.

Good Samaritans often are found standing in the wings waiting God's next assignment. That was the case for committee member Judi Harris, Ph.D. Judi guided me formally in class but then was a willing servant of His in her repeated and patient explanations of qualitative methods of research. Whether coaching me for my qualifying exams, debriefing a field experience, or playing "devil's advocate, " Judi was an asset to me. Thank you, Judi, for being my teacher, my friend, my coach, and finally my committee member.

There remains one indefatigable person who with patience and perseverance steadfastly guided and oared me through deep waters. The ingenuous one who was always open and sincere and expressed her concerns for me by her every action. The incomparable one who in her matchless wisdom and superlative care watched over me like a mother hen. The incalculable one whose multitudinous talents were extended to me in incomputable ways and who kept me on the road to victory. The erudite one whose brilliance was a daily inspiration to me to press on to my goal. The irrefutable one whose knowledge and strong will left me no doubt but that I could attain my goal. The irresistible one whose indomitable spirit lifted me when it seemed that I could not go on. The irreplaceable one who has been my mentor, my motivator, my friend, and the Good Samaritan who did so much for me to make graduation day happen: my dissertation committee supervisor, Diane L. Schallert, Ph.D., is all the above and I am accordingly indescribably grateful to her.

I could not conclude accolades without including Jessye Ley Cleveland, my medical service dog. Jessye not only provided medical aid, and often attended class with me, but entertained me daily and was always happy to see me on good days and bad.

If there are any who read these acknowledgments and think them too long, may I remind you that my whole life is qualitative, just as my research has been! I would have no credentials entitling me to write these pages at all; I would have no particular insights to share into how motivations enable us to overcome, if it had not been for the incredible provisions described in these admittedly lengthy pages of praises!

At the time of the accident in 1984, many said recovering was impossible. Impossibilities are God's opportunities through Good Samaritans. A brass plaque was mounted to the dash in the Mercedes bearing the inscription of Isaiah 40:31. This same verse is woven into a tapestry, which hangs in my entry hall, and I read it several times each day. Being the recipient of such grace, sustained all this way by His host of Good Samaritans, both named and unnamed, has taught me a deep appreciation of this verse:

> But they that wait upon the Lord shall renew their strength, they shall mount up with wings as eagles, they shall run and not be weary, they shall walk and not faint. Isaiah 40:31

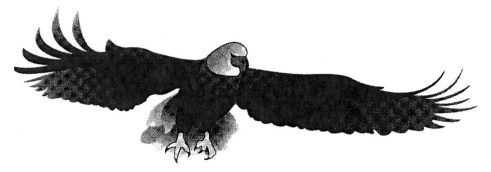

To God be the Glory great things He hath done!

Momentum: A Model for Motivation in Rehabilitation for Individuals with Traumatic Brain Injury

Publication No._____

Lynda Gail Cleveland, Ph.D.

The University of Texas at Austin, 1998

Supervisor: Diane Lemonnier Schallert

Every year millions of traumatic brain injuries (TBI) caused by any type of sudden external force upon the head occur in the United States, accompanied by a range of complex physical, cognitive, behavioral, and emotional problems. The period of time between injury and re-adaptation to social roles is generally labeled rehabilitation as the survivor works to achieve recovery of function. A phenomenon that has stumped the medical community for decades, and still remains unsolved is how best to foster recovery for TBI individuals, although there is general agreement that "motivation" plays a key role. This study was designed to address the following research question: What is the genesis and nature of the motivation experienced by individuals with TBI in rehabilitation? I sought to understand the motivational factors and to generate a model of these factors grounded in the data.

The phenomenological approach of grounded theory was used to examine the experiences of individuals with TBI as they constructed meaning from events and interactions in their rehabilitation setting.

The research was conducted at a large rehabilitation facility specializing in recovery from traumatic brain injury. I served as a student/intern at this facility during the nine months of data gathering. In addition to being a participant-observer working closely with 64 TBI clients, I gathered data from archival documents (client medical records and progress reports) and conducted one-on-one interviews with clients, selected family members, and staff members. Data were analyzed using open, axial, and selective coding processes prior to selecting the central phenomenon for the study.

For individuals with TBI in this study, the outcome of motivation was *engagement* in rehabilitation programs. The data in this study suggested that participation was achieved as a result of a synergy that was interactionally created by four contextual categories: one's *perception of self, perception of recovery, vision,* and *personal interactions.* This synergy was called *momentum*, the central phenomenon. These categories are presented metaphorically in a gyroscopic model. Momentum generated continued rehabilitation participation, that, in turn, enabled the client to return to community life at the highest level possible.

Table of Contents

List of Tables

List of Figures

CHAPTER 1

INTRODUCTION

"I don't let people into my world. I didn't want to let you into my world until I learned you had TBI [traumatic brain injury]. Then I wanted to know you better."

-Terri, Tallangatta client

Background

Prior to this study, my professional experience was focused in three areas: educator, stage/video director, and motivational speaker. My experience spanned three decades, and involved hundreds of students at the secondary as well as university levels, uncounted thousands of individuals in audiences across three continents, and hundreds of actors and technicians in stage and video productions. These situations demanded that I not only teach, but that I also motivate. I never really pondered the question of what motivation was, as it appeared to me that motivation was a contagious by-product of my own enthusiasm. In the classroom, the types of motivation such as intrinsic, extrinsic, expectancy-value, or needs-based, never consciously entered into my goal-setting strategies with students. During the decade that I taught in the public school classroom, I also participated in the creation of medical educational programs for large city hospitals. As my experience broadened over the years, my focus turned to medical education. My new students were individuals with illness or injury. Even though these students, who were patients, participated and seemed interested in the content I was presenting, they often did not use the knowledge or skills they were taught. I soon

1

realized I needed to understand more fully what triggered motivation so that I could develop programs and situations that would impact students' (patients') use of the knowledge and skills they learned. So, I sought to identify the triggers of motivation and turned to professionals in the medical field: physicians, nurses, technicians, and educators. The more individuals I asked, the more varied the answers I received. Everyone seemed to know exactly what motivation was until they had to verbalize a definition. "Yes, motivation is.... ah," "well, you know, the energy, uh, well, hmmm...," "well, following treatment plans...uh...," "that feeling you get inside when you want to do something..uh...." were the common answers I received.

Motivation, it seemed, was defined in terms of patient compliance with medical advice. From the definitions I received, motivation was that something that triggered whether one's behavior worked toward or away from compliance with recommended clinical regimes. While the issue of what triggered motivation continued to haunt me, I tucked the motivation phenomenon in my memory as curious and undefinable.

I was first introduced to traumatic brain injury in 1984 in Melbourne, Australia. I was a front-seat passenger in a Mercedes that was hit head on by an out-of-control 14 ton flat-bed truck. Although I was critically injured, the grace of God and the mechanical wizardry of Mercedes spared my life. At the time of my accident, I was a successful businesswoman, traveling internationally, and with a life planned with a wonderful man. Therefore, my premorbid life had been most positive and rewarding.

After several weeks in the hospital following the accident, I was discharged home for "bed rest and outpatient rehabilitation therapy." According to my medical records, I had physical therapy, as well as occupational and speech therapy. I recall weeks running into months and years of agonizing physical therapy. Just as vivid as my memory of the pain of physical therapy, I remember the frustration of being told, "You've changed," "You'll never work again," "You are not the same person." Entries into my medical records indicate these are accurate memories, "…it would appear that she has undergone a personality change…" (1987). "Overall, her long-term prognosis is not good" (1988).

> Lynda continues to experience spells with a loss of consciousness, incontinence, convulsive movements of limbs…there is confusion of her use of words …(1991).

> Lynda requires continuous, round-the-clock nursing support, she is incapable of independent living, there is no way she will be capable of supporting herself financially in the foreseeable future, and she will need to be on medication and medical supervision for a long time to come (1992).

I struggled to rediscover who I was by working in a hospital as a videographer, by writing a book about overcoming trauma called *Detour Ahead* (Cleveland & Taylor, 1985); yet nothing seemed to return the old "me." I experienced extreme mood swings and emotional outbursts. I looked in the mirror and did not know who it was staring back at me. The things I thought were certainly different from the things I did; my body and mind seemed to be out of synchronization.

I was fortunate; I had a tremendous foundation of support from family and friends both in Australia and America. In spite of this support network, I was riding a roller coaster of emotions and personal changes. I always assumed I would be "well" after my discharge from the hospital. Despite my dreams and wishes for "wellness," my physical injuries healed yet my brain functioning capabilities continued to progress at a very slow pace. I had suffered a rather severe traumatic brain injury. I would have to learn to live with it for the rest of my life.

In spite of the story that unfolded through 1991, the events since 1992 and beyond perhaps speak the loudest about motivation. In 1992, I was medically cleared to attempt community reentry under close supervision. I still required nursing assistance; I was not cleared to drive; and I was not capable of total independent living; yet, I attempted to return to school to upgrade my abilities in order to be competitive in the workforce. The internal driving force that had always pushed me to strive to be the very best I could seemed to drive me even harder now.

As I reflect upon those first two years back in the real world, the community, and an academic environment, I recall experiences that emotionally drained me, laughing one minute and crying the next. I have to chuckle as I recall the notes plastered about my house in order to remember simple things like locking the door, unplugging the coffee pot, and completing a dressing sequence in the proper order. On the flip side of this humor, memories of my experiences can again move me to tears, and I taste the hurt of being shunned in public, or being in a room full of people and feeling all alone, or living with the "silent epidemic." Traumatic brain injury is called the "silent epidemic" (Zitney, 1995) because it occurs in the lives of so many individuals, yet is so misunderstood by those on the outside. It hurts to recall the frustration of asking for help and being

4

told, "Why is that a problem? You look normal. You should have no problem with this assignment…everyone has problems in this course; you can work it out." I began to sense inadequacies in the rehabilitation systems that failed to teach compensatory strategies for life beyond head injury. My experiences have shown me the fallacy in the common belief that after 18 months or so an individual suffering from traumatic brain injury has made as much progress as can be expected.

When asked about the TBI rehabilitation practices, Seaton, executive director of a large rehabilitation facility, once commented, "individuals with disabilities do not plateau, but environments do, and progress is based on learning" (1997). His belief was that an individual suffering from TBI does not reach a certain point in recovery then level out or quit; rather it is the rehabilitation environment around him/her that peaks and offers a less challenging and stimulating environment for recovery. To progress, an individual with TBI must be learning. Learning requires rehabilitation programs that are stimulating teaching environments.

I am testimony to this philosophy. I was placed in a rehabilitation program filled with constant activity, encouragement to return to work, and constant instruction. My rehabilitation caregivers all classified me as a "motivated patient." Why? I have been fortunate to continue to progress in my rehabilitation journeys, but what characteristics were present that caused my motivation to surface and continue? Why did my motivation not wane? Why did I follow recommendations for self-care, while other individuals did not comply with their medical instructions? My personal traumatic brain injury experience coupled with my experience in trying to motivate patients to comply with their self-care plans seemed to come together as a natural research opportunity.

Rationale

Rationale for this study comes from several lines of literature that are reviewed in greater detail in Chapter 2. Here I present brief highlights.

TRAUMATIC BRAIN INJURY INCIDENCE

Every year, millions of head injuries occur in the United States. Bumps on the head are ubiquitous in human activity and, therefore, the incidence of head injury is difficult to ascertain. Hospitalization is the most common way of identifying the frequency of head injury. Annually, the estimated number of individuals sustaining injury to the brain, representing all levels of severity, ranges between 500,000 to 1.5 million, with approximately 500,000 requiring hospitalization (Parker, 1990). Approximately 50,000 – 70,000 injuries are classified moderate to severe; these individuals will live with a combination of cognitive, physical, behavioral, and/or emotional deficits and will require some or continual rehabilitation for the rest of their normal life-span (Seaton, ed., 1997).

The brain can be injured internally from illnesses such as stroke, tumor, Parkinson's disease or Alzheimer's Disease; however, the injuries that are the subject of this study are those of a traumatic nature: those caused by a sudden external force upon the head. The probability for head injury is greater (2 times) for men than women; the peak incidence for injury is between 15 and 24 years of age (Kraus & Sorenson, 1994). The majority of traumatic brain injuries are due to motor vehicle or pedestrian injuries, work-related accidents, falls, assaults, and suicide attempts (Seaton, ed., 1997).

TRAUMATIC BRAIN INJURY RESEARCH

The brain is our most complex and vulnerable organ. The brain is the operations center and network coordinator for who we are, the way we think, the way we feel, and the way we act. One traumatic brain injury (TBI) survivor expressed an injury to the brain as "an insult to our being–ness…" (Sharon, online). The brain does, indeed, control our "being–ness," all voluntary and involuntary movements, actions, and thoughts. An injury to the brain can change everything about us in a matter of seconds.

A range of complex physical, cognitive, behavioral, and emotional problems define the nature of traumatic brain injury (TBI). The period of time between injury and readaptation to social roles is generally labeled rehabilitation as the survivor works to achieve recovery of function. A phenomenon that has stumped the medical community for decades, and, to date, remains unsolved is the puzzle of how best to foster recovery for the traumatically brain injured patient. About the only brain fact agreed upon by all researchers is that the brain is the one organ that defies any absolutes of how it will or will not relate to injury or illness. While the injury or illness itself may have common defining characteristics, the ultimate effect upon the individual will manifest itself differently in each case

(Goldstein, 1952; Haffey & Lewis, 1989; Prigatano, 1989; Prigatano, Pepping & Klonoff, 1986; Stern, 1996).

In recent years, strict medical emphasis when discussing traumatic brain injuries has shifted to include a discussion of the psychological as well as the physiological aspects of recovery. Research focused upon the relationship of the brain and behavior recognizes that the affective elements such as emotions and motivations are most influential, however difficult to define and therefore not discussed in detail in formal reports (Cahn, 1997; Cicerone, 1989; Davis, 1990; Davies, 1994; Persinger, 1993; Simkins, 1994).

Experts in the field generally agree upon three broad categories of deficits following injury to the brain:

- personality and behavioral impairments,
- cognitive impairments,
- physical impairments (Cahn, 1997).

Likewise, there seems to be agreement on the keys to rehabilitation for the TBI patient: medical stability, followed by the presence of a support team, time, and finally, the TBIer's effort or "motivation." Those assisting TBI survivors need to agree upon individuals' goals for themselves:

- to live, work, and enjoy life,
- to redevelop social and family relationships,
- to participate within the community (Senelick and Ryan, 1991).

During his term as President of the United States, George Bush declared the 1990's the *Decade of the Brain*. During this decade, greater attention has been paid to rehabilitation research, trends, and techniques for individuals suffering a traumatic brain injury. Many treatment programs have purported to apply specialized techniques that will remediate both cognitive and behavioral deficits of TBI survivors. In the literature on rehabilitation techniques as discussed in Chapter 2, a discussion of motivation and the effect motivation has upon TBI survivors are presented as if everyone agreed on what it is. There seems to be an intuitive feeling for "motivation," and yet it escapes absolute definition. I find it ironic that in scientific fields such as general medicine and rehabilitation, a force that cannot be defined nor scientifically measured in order to substantiate or prove its value is acknowledged as one of the strongest elements necessary for rehabilitation or recovery.

As discussed in Chapter 2, the Health Belief Model and the PRECEDE (Preceding, Reinforcing, Enabling Causes in Educational Diagnosis and Evaluation) model are two of the more popular instruments used in rehabilitation to indicate the motivational tendencies of the individual. However, neither of these instruments offer *how* or *why* motivation occurs. Therefore, I turned to the educational psychology literature of motivation and learning for guidance in discovering the keys to motivation.

MOTIVATION

According to Petri (1991), "motivation is the concept we use when we describe the forces acting on or within an organism to initiate and direct behavior" (p. 3). Motivation is typically measured through inference. We can infer that motivation has orchestrated action when changes in response follow changes in stimulus conditions. A decade ago there were over 100 definitions of motivation

9

(Kleinginna and Kleinginna, 1981) and while there is no consensus on one single definition, motivation is typified with three characteristics. These three activities are observable in the production of behavior.

- Usually there is *overt action* in a particular direction that can be seen and often measured, such as the number of steps taken for the individual with TBI.

- The second characteristic often noted is *persistence.* The longer an individual persists to accomplish a task or reach a goal, the greater the motivation.

- The third commonly agreed upon characteristic is that of *vigor*, which is energy in response to the goal, such as rehabilitation (Petri, 1991, p. 4-6).

Nearly every journal or text related to brain research offers the term motivation in the index and offers discussions on one of the above three characteristics. Disappointing to the practitioner or researcher, however, is that the entry is usually a very short mention of emotion or motivation developed only to the level of simply recognizing the importance of the topic. Rarely does this progress to a full discussion or analysis of the concept (c.f., Ostwald, 1989; Prigatano, 1990).

Because neither the educational nor rehabilitation literature effectively solve the riddle of what triggered and sustained motivation, I sought to integrate the fields to create the theoretical framework for this study. Interpersonal relationships in these two fields are similar in their interactional qualities, such as teacher-to-student and doctor-to-patient; parent-teacher conferences and family-health care team conferences; and low/high achieving students and low/high achieving patients. The literature on motivation in the classroom, while often examining motivation in light of the dichotomy of intrinsic and extrinsic aspects, acknowledges that there are innumerable combinations that energize an individual (Reeve, 1996). The rehabilitation literature offers multiple factors influencing recovery. Each of these two fields, education and rehabilitation, point to such factors as one's environment, demographics, culture, and family background to illustrate the multiple factors influencing motivation. However, it seemed to me that the link I noted most often was that of the learner characteristics of the individual. The educational as well as rehabilitation literature emphasizes the importance of understanding the learner and what influences him/her.

LEARNING

The environmental factors mentioned led me to look to the literature on learning and change that has explored the role of the social environment in the construction of comprehension (e.g. Kress, 1989; Shotter, 1993; Wells, 1987; Vygotsky, 1994) because it offered theoretical constructs useful for describing how contextual factors interact with an individual's experience. With the knowledge that shared experiences do affect the progress of individuals with traumatic brain injuries, an understanding of socially constructed knowledge as defined by Prawat and Floden (1994, p. 40) as is "created from a shared rather than an individual experience," was seen to be appropriate for this study. Likewise, because so much of the growth and progress of an individual with TBI is based upon his/her learning, the psychological processes involved in learning were also important.

Preliminary Studies

In the year preceding this study, two preliminary studies were conducted and are discussed in detail in Chapter 3. These studies served to establish the parameters for the present research effort. As one result of the two preliminary studies, the guiding question for this inquiry focuses on the personal as well as societal elements that seemed to enhance or erode participants' actions taken toward recovery. Nearly any rehabilitation text about TBI identifies the downfalls, but omits the activators of progress leaving unaddressed what triggers motivation.

Statement of Problem/Purpose

What, then, is the key to assisting the individual with a traumatic brain injury (TBI) to make the greatest progress possible? With the numbers of individuals suffering brain injury in the United States increasing, the need to motivate survivors to work at their rehabilitation efforts is paramount. Therefore, this study was designed to address the following research question:

What is the genesis and nature of motivation experienced by patients with a traumatic brain injury in rehabilitation?

Methods

An individual's dream for recovery from a traumatic brain injury is intertwined with his/her beliefs, values, dreams, attitudes, remaining functionality, and support structure. According to Lincoln (1992), all these characteristics form a part of what we label culture. The cultural and social aspects of life are "ill 3understood using conventional inquiry but are well researched in all their complexity using the means and the methods of the field anthropologist" (Lincoln, 1992, p. 388). Therefore, I chose to use qualitative methods and constructivist philosophy to explore my research question. While this approach represented a shift from health research's tradition of collecting hard quantitative data, it offered the power of exploring behavior, interactivity, belief systems, and meaning given to events as seen from the perspectives of the TBI population. The data gathered in this fashion can be complementary, synergistic, and reinforcing the traditional research results. One of the greatest needs in health research is more study of human beings enacting health practices in homes, schools, and work sites (Lincoln, 1992). In her assessment of the need for qualitative medical research, Lincoln (1992) cited Tony Kuzel:

> ...the medical literature on health promotion/disease prevention is long on ideas and systems and short on 'grounded theory,' i.e., theory which is generated by systematic observation of community-based clinical practice and which is corroborated by the characters in that practice...(p. 387)

The particular approach to qualitative research taken in this study was grounded theory as presented by Strauss and Corbin (1990). In the following sections, I discuss the characteristics of my study: the methods, the participants, the process of data gathering, and the participant-observer.

13

QUALITATIVE METHODS

Qualitative research is "any kind of research that produces findings not arrived at by the means of statistical procedures or other means of quantification" (Strauss & Corbin, 1990, p. 17). Research of this nature can be about topics such as individuals' lives, behavior, stories, social movements, or relationships. According to Strauss and Corbin, the three major components of qualitative research are:

- data, with interviews and observations the most common types,
- analytic or interpretative procedures for conceptualizing data's meaning,
- written and verbal reports.

In the tradition of grounded theory, a theory or model of influences on a phenomenon is inductively derived from the study of the situation or phenomenon it represents. Thus, the goal of this study was to build a theory of motivation for traumatic brain injury (TBI) survivors in a rehabilitation center. Methodological recommendations by Strauss and Corbin (1990) were followed. Data collection, analysis, and theory stand in reciprocal relationships with each other. I did not begin with a theory and attempt to prove it. Rather, I began with an area of study and allowed a theory to emerge as a by-product of data generation and interpretation. The analysis I did was comprised of three major types of coding: open coding (labeling data), axial coding (categorizing data), and selective coding (interpreting and validating data) (Strauss & Corbin, 1990). I also created a conditional matrix coding (Strauss & Corbin, 1990), analytical framework for

14

studying relationships, as I built my theory. These steps are discussed in more detail in Chapter 4.

PARTICIPANTS

I selected individuals recovering from a traumatic brain injury (TBI) as the focus for this study because I had personal experience in this field. All participants were survivors of a traumatic brain injury (TBI), that is, a sudden external blow to the head. The majority of the participants were victims of motor vehicle or work-related accidents. All were hospitalized for at least three days with a diagnosis of either open or closed head injury. All participants had a passing grade of 75% on the Galveston Orientation and Awareness Test at the time of this study. Early medical indicators such as the Glasgow Coma Scale or the Rancho Los Amigos Scale were noted when available for possible future correlation with recovery perceptions, however, these descriptive data were not considered when selecting participants. Both men and women survivors form the sample. Participants were from varied ethnic backgrounds and were between 18-52 years of age. Individuals with a premorbid history of drug or alcohol abuse or mental disorders such as manic depression or schizophrenia were not considered. Medical records were studied for indications of premorbid personalities so that correlations between premorbid states and perceptions of recovery could be uncovered, but these were not selection criteria. All participants were residents at a large facility that specializes in the rehabilitation and community reintegration of TBI survivors.

In addition to the TBI participants, several support members were interviewed including family members as well as therapists involved with the individuals. I served as a participant observer at the research sites. Due to the qualitative nature of this study and the inductive process of building a theory of motivation in TBI recovery, there were no preconceived limitations upon the number of study participants. In the end, the total number of active participants was 64, representing the number with whom I had direct, regular contact. To protect the identity of each participant, whether client, family, or staff, all names used in this dissertation are pseudonyms. There are also occasions where the characteristics of several clients and staff personnel are combined to create one illustrative client.

PROCESS OF DATA GATHERING

As a participant observer, I worked as a staff member at the rehabilitation center for nine months. During this time, I observed the clients in every aspect of their day, including interactions, personal struggles and triumphs. I conducted semi-structured interviews on several occasions, and periodically I debriefed with various rehabilitation personnel to check the accuracy of my findings. The guiding questions for this study, discussed in Chapter 4, focused on both the intrinsic and extrinsic factors that seemed to energize the clients to action, or conversely, to stop the action. The daily activities of the participants were recorded in my field notes in addition to often being audio-recorded. Both forms of these data were then transcribed. In addition to these sources of data, I conducted semi-structured interviews with most of the clients. At times these interviews were conducted while the client and I worked one-on-one completing daily tasks such as physical exercises. At other times, these interviews occurred during a one-on-one prearranged meeting time, and others were conducted in a group setting. All interviews were audio-recorded and later transcribed. All made use of the guiding foci detailed in Chapter 4. In addition to these data sources, I studied medical records, institutional records, and personal artifacts including daily journals, of the participants. In each of these cases, the data I felt to be pertinent to the discovery of motivational factors were recorded in my field notes for later transcription. In addition to the data generated with the clients, casual interviews were conducted with staff and family members when opportunities presented themselves. The final source of data was the Future Time Perspective questionnaire, also discussed in Chapter 4 and included in Appendix A.

RESEARCHER AS PARTICIPANT OBSERVER

As noted by Lincoln (1992), the strength of a paradigm for inquiry is also its weakness. That statement holds true also for the benefits of participant observation, especially for one who is personally involved. I strongly believe that my own personal experiences of the last 13 years were a great contributor to my understanding of the struggles and perceptions of the participants. There is no question that my experience with TBI allowed me to enjoy a close camaraderie with participants in daily activities, failures, and triumphs. The nature of these relationships allowed me the privilege of more in-depth, personal conversations, interviews, and questioning on issues that those of us having sustained a brain injury do not readily discuss or share with "outsiders."

However, realizing that this very strength can also be a weakness, I made two major provisions, educational and emotional, to assure that my participants would only be positive benefactors of my bias. In order to protect the safety of all participants, I completed the basic staff education course required by all staff working with clients at the research facilities. Basic first aid techniques, medications, seizure control, and behavior management skills were some of the topics covered in this introductory staff training. Training continued throughout the research project in the form of participation in the Certified Brain Injury Specialist training programs, allowing even greater competency both working with individuals with brain injury, and in my ability to recognize accurately what I was seeing in their progress. In addition to the training, I passed all physical examinations, drug screens, and criminal investigations conducted by the participating facilities. I also took emotional precautions by scheduling weekly, often daily, debriefing sessions with Barbara Holmes, a Ph.D., R.N. colleague, my dissertation supervisor, and a close personal friend. By having a release for my emotional experience, often reliving my own days in rehabilitation, I attempted to distance myself emotionally when working with my participants.

Conclusion

This dissertation is organized in six chapters. Following this chapter is a discussion of the literature that first influenced this study. Chapter 3 is a review of the findings in the two preliminary studies conducted. The qualitative methods used in the present study are detailed in the methods chapter. In presenting the results in Chapter 5, I attempted to offer "thick [extremely detailed] descriptions" (Lincoln & Guba, 1985) of phenomena and their contextual settings to support my emerging theoretical model. Chapter 6 discusses the findings from this study in relationship to the context of the literature of motivation.

CHAPTER 2

REVIEW OF LITERATURE

"I thought I couldn't read these big books. I actually learned something by reading this book and the pictures helped. This is great. I like this new job. I feel better in myself."

-Todd, Windy Hill client

Introduction

During the 1990s, proclaimed the *Decade of the Brain* by the Bush administration, there has been a proliferation of traumatic brain injury (TBI) rehabilitation literature (e.g., Armstrong, 1991; Ashley & Krych, eds., 1995; Crisp, 1994; Ellerd, et. al, 1994; Kreutzer & Wehman, eds., 1990; Senelick & Ryan, 1991; Willer, et. al, 1991). The importance of motivation was noted or implied in most of the TBI rehabilitation literature reviewed. However, motivation has never really been defined or discussed in depth. Therefore, the design of this study was to generate a theory of motivation from observations and interviews of survivors of traumatic brain injury, their family members, and professionals specializing in TBI rehabilitation.

In order to accomplish this task, theoretical frameworks were borrowed from neurology and neurological rehabilitation literature as well as from the literature on classroom research and educational psychology, including the study of motivation and learning. This review of literature provides a discussion of the initial framework that provided the theoretical basis for this study. This investigation focuses on the interrelationships of three topics: (1) rehabilitation,

(2) motivation, and (3) learning. By investigating the interrelationships of these topics, I hoped to capture the nature of motivation as it relates to the survivor of a TBI. This review of literature is not intended to provide detailed research in any of these areas, but rather to offer a broad background in the areas that provide an underpinning for this study. The understanding of the foundations for this study will not be enhanced by a review of all the literature analyzed; however, the reader may find some of the sources beneficial, though they were not cited. Therefore, a complete listing of all works that were a major influence on this study have been included in the bibliography. The review is presented in three sections: rehabilitation, motivation, and learning.

Research in Rehabilitation from Traumatic Brain Injury

OVERVIEW

A specialty field for the rehabilitation of survivors of traumatic brain injury (TBI) emerged in the late 1970s (Ashley & Krych, 1995). The TBI rehabilitation industry was largely recognized only by private organizations financially responsible for the costs of the care for TBI survivors. The costs were considerable and most rehabilitation facilities were not equipped to deal with the long-term care most often required. Survival rates following traumatic brain injury (TBI) had increased largely due to helicopter evacuation and medical advances. Helicopter evacuation, introduced for the care of military personnel in the Vietnam and Korean wars, enabled quick transportation to specialized trauma centers as well as rapid pre-hospital stabilization. Dramatic advances in diagnosis, neurosurgery, neuroanatomy, neurophysiology, and neuropharmacology skills also improved the survival rates (Bontke, 1990; Browning in Ashley & Krych, 1995). Based on rising survival rates of those with traumatic brain injury (TBI), the number of TBI rehabilitation facilities has increased exponentially from the late 1970s and early 1980s. The Brain Injury Association of America (formerly the National Head Injury Foundation) noted fewer than three dozen dedicated head injury programs in 1980, a count that grew to over 700 by the end of the decade. The disability rights movement of the 1970s, culminating with the Rehabilitation Act of 1973, altered the image of individuals with disabilities from one of a medical burden to society to one of a group deserving socio-political rights. In this movement, individuals with disabilities actively sought to redefine their image of independence (Pfeiffer, 1993).

In 1985, the National Head Injury Foundation entered into a cooperative agreement with the United States Office of Special Education and Rehabilitation Services, the Council of State Administrators of Vocational Rehabilitation, and the National Association of State Directors of Special Education to recognize traumatic brain injury as a specific disability. The lack of public attention to this major cause of death and disability and the lack of public funding for the treatment of brain injured persons caused the Brain Injury Association (formerly The National Head Injury Foundation) to call TBI "the silent epidemic." In 1990, the Americans with Disabilities Act (ADA) solidified the rights of disabled Americans with the decree that individuals with disabilities were not be discriminated against in employment, transportation, communication, or access to public facilities. The ADA also granted the right to these individuals to request reasonable accommodations and to defend themselves in a court of law against discriminatory treatment (Sachs & Redd, 1993).

Since the early 1970s and the increasing focus on the individuals with disabilities, there has been an escalation of research studies on various components of head injury rehabilitation. Prior to the 1980s, the survivor of a TBI was faced with debilitating physical, cognitive, emotional, social, communicative, and behavioral deficits. Because of the aforementioned deficits, society tended to apply negative labels to those surviving TBI. Until recent years, the individual with a TBI faced complications of conditions that were difficult to define medically and perplexing socially. The disabilities from TBI were more complex and resistant to rehabilitation efforts than other brain injuries; therefore, treatment was often a perplexing challenge. The literature in the last 20 years on traumatic brain injury (TBI) speaks to the ramifications of and recovery from TBI from three points of view: neuroscientific implications, rehabilitation practices, and medical jurisprudence. Each of these aforementioned areas offers discussions on problems caused by deficits in motivation after injury; however, none of the areas offers a solution.

NEUROSCIENTIFIC IMPLICATIONS

A daunting experience waits any individual attempting to categorize relationships of post-morbid TBI behavior to specific injury and brain region function. In the field of traumatic brain injury research, there has been a battle fought on the specificity of where and how a damaged brain will manifest itself in emotional and motivational behavior. The focus of this study is not of a neurobiological nature; however, an appreciation of the neuropathology of TBI and the neuroscientific arguments is beneficial to understanding the research foundations of this project.

"[Traumatic] brain injury is an insult to the brain, not of a degenerative or congenital nature, that may produce cognitive, behavioral, emotional, or physical deficits. These impairments are usually permanent and result in partial or total disability." (Seaton, ed., 1997). Open-head injuries (skull is penetrated) tend to be more localized than closed-head injuries (sudden external blow to the skull). Closed-head injuries (CHI) are the most common of all craniocerebral traumas (Rosenthal et. al, 1990). Usually the damaging force in CHI is that of the impact itself, such as an acceleration/deceleration impact sustained in a motor vehicle accident. This type of impact causes a coup (point of impact)/contracoup (opposite point of impact) injury to the brain (Golden, et.al, 1983). Both primary and secondary neuropathological insults can occur to the brain in injury. White matter is sheared—one part of the brain moved at a different speed than surrounding tissues, stretching the fibers—resulting in direct structural damage, while edema, hematomas, and hypoxia may account for secondary damage (Prigatano, 1986). The functional units of the human brain are constantly interacting with one another. The outermost section of the brain is that of the cerebral cortex, which is divided into two hemispheres connected by a large bundle of neural fibers for transfer of information. The functions of the left cerebral hemisphere are primarily language, including reading, writing, listening, and speaking. The right cerebral hemisphere specializes in non-language or

24

spatial abilities such as recognizing and solving puzzles, drawing pictures, or knowing directions. The cortex is anatomically divided into four lobes: frontal, parietal, temporal, and occipital (Seaton, ed., 1997).

Subcortical structures (brain stem, cerebellum, thalamus, basal ganglia, and limbic system) are located beneath the cortex and play a vital role in regulating affective behavior. The cortical and subcortical systems function in an integrated fashion for the expression of emotions and motivation (Parker, 1990). The neural pathways connecting the subcortical structures with the cortex play a vital role in affective behavior. These pathways are often damaged in TBI.

The vulnerability of the tips of the frontal lobe, temporal lobe, and the brain-stem structures have been the emphasis of the traditional views of the neuropathology of closed-head injury (CHI) due to the position of the human brain in the skull (Levin, Benton, & Grossman, 1983). However, research shows that there are many types of damage from brain injuries. For example, in addition to shearing damage, hemorrhage, or ischemic damage is possible, which often affects the basal ganglia and hippocampal structure. (Graham, Adams, and Doyle, 1978). Therefore, survivors of TBI frequently have memory, emotion, and motivation problems that appear to have a clear organic origin (Prigatano, 1986). The frustrating outcome from the neuroscientific literature is that of the recognition of the importance of motivation, the multiple biological descriptions of its origin, and no practical guidelines for encouraging or reestablishing the motivational drive for the survivor of TBI. From the multitude of descriptions, I have selected only three entries discussing the organic origins of motivation for examples of this literature.

Example 1:

While it is unlikely that a specific (i.e., focal) brain lesion will produce a specific personality disturbance, different lesions may influence various neurophysiological and neuropsychological substrates of emotion and motivation in a predictable manner. Some lesions will influence arousal and attentional mechanisms, others will influence the cognitive appraisal of feeling states and the manner in which feelings are expressed (Prigatano, 1986, p. 49).

Example 2:

While there has been much written about motivational systems, knowledge of their anatomic and physiologic bases is far from complete …

it is important to note that motivational behavior appears to be mediated by diencephalic limbic-cortex networks.

Although the anatomic and physiologic basis for the right hemisphere's special role in intentional activity is unknown, the limbic system, which plays a critical role in motivation, has two major outputs to the cortex, one from the hippocampus and the other via the cingulate gyrus…(Levin, Eisenberg, & Benton, 1991, p. 209).

Example 3:

The hypothalamus is often grouped with the thalamus as constituting the diencephalon. The hypothalamus appears to be involved in motivation, and the amygdala appears to have a role in emotion; clearly, both factors affect what we remember. (Kosslyn & Koenig, 1992, p.345).

While most researchers agree on the organic source of motivated behavior, the limbic system interaction with the lobes, there are those who oppose the organic explanation:

As is the case with attention, lack of motivation is not caused by damage to some hypothetical center in the brain as is sometimes supposed. Motivation is very much a by-product of the patient's environment and the way in which he/she is helped to achieve realistic goals. (Davies, 1994, p. 19).

There has not been much to operationalize our understanding of motivation with specific tips for the survivor or those assisting him/her with sustaining motivation long enough to achieve results. Prigatano, perhaps, offers the most workable explanation for the rehabilitation specialist:

> Personality is defined as patterns of emotional and motivational responses that develop over the life of the organism; are highly influenced by early life experiences; are modifiable, but not easily changed, by behavioral or teaching methods; and greatly influence (and are influenced by) cognitive processes . . .the form of a given emotional and/or motivational response is highly dependent on the environmental consequences as well as the biological state of the organism…As such, biological, psychological, and psychosocial constructs are inevitably involved in defining personality.

> If feelings can be considered the basic representation for homeostatic states of the organism, the terms emotion and motivation can be used to refer to more complex and refined feelings states that incorporate the basic homeostasis but also go beyond it. Motivation refers to the complex feeling states that parallel hierarchical goal-seeking behavior (Simon, 1967). As such, it can be described as the arousal component of behavior which sees to it that a plan of action is developed and executed.

> These considerations have two important corollaries …First, disturbances in brain-stem and related structures may influence basic arousal and/or attentional mechanisms…. Second, disturbances of higher "cerebral" or "cortical" centers may influence the ability of the person to perceive and interpret correctly feelings in self and others. These emotional and motivational disturbances flow not from a lack of sustained or modulated arousal but from an inability to deal cognitively with arousal-producing stimuli. (Prigatano, 1986, p. 31-32).

Thus, while the neurophysiological substrates of motivation were defined through research, operationally (that is day-to-day functioning) was not defined. The sequelae of a TBI proved to be far more complicated and the disabilities more extensive than similar populations (Ashley & Krych, eds., 1995). Injuries to the brain (especially CHI) are generally of a diffuse nature, consequently manifesting themselves in complex combinations of post acute challenges. While injuries to the brain may be of similar location and type, no two individuals ever experience exactly the same outcome due to factors such as premorbid characteristics, or financial as well as personal resources (e.g., Ashley & Krych, 1995; Crisp, 1992; Heilman & Valenstein, 1993; Kaplan, 1993; Senelick & Ryan, 1991).

Prigatano (1988) summarizes the dilemma of the neuroscientific organic knowledge of motivation without the operational knowledge:

> In summary, emotional and motivational disturbances are common after traumatic brain injury and may be crucial determinants for functional recovery. These dimensions influence how an individual will engage in rehabilitation programs. They also impact on how the patient adapts to higher cerebral deficits. Emotional and motivational problems have not figured prominently in any major theory of recovery of function. This appears to be in part because these two concepts have not been adequately defined and are not easily investigated in highly controlled ways. Both include an arousal component that can have reinforcing qualities. (Prigatano, 1978, p. 348.)

Craniocerebral trauma has a major impact on the psychological, social, and vocational aspects of an individual. While these changes are difficult to understand scientifically, clinical manifestations are predictable.

REHABILITATION PRACTICES

The ultimate goal in the rehabilitation of any injury is the return of the patient to his/her ability to again function as an independent human being. Because changes in cognitive functioning and disorders of personality occur frequently in the TBI survivor, there is a major psychosocial adjustment for the survivor and his/her family (Prigatano, 1986). Rehabilitation for the TBI survivor is divided, as is the literature, into neurological recovery, discussed above, and social recovery. "Social" recovery encompasses the recovery of physical, communicative, cognitive, and emotional functions after the neurological recovery has been completed (Ashley & Krych, 1995). Individuals sustaining a traumatic brain injury each arrive with varied significant life experiences. These experiences are crucial to the development of a rehabilitation program and impact the rehabilitative process. The current literature on rehabilitative efforts can be divided into six major areas of concentration: neuropsychological issues, rehabilitation program trends, family matters, self-awareness, medical jurisprudence, and compliance.

Neuropsychological Issues

The study of higher cerebral deficits following traumatic brain injury has used neurological criteria for its scientific investigations. For example, various correlations have been made with the TBI patients' post-traumatic amnesia (PTA) base as the primary predictor. Such comparisons have been made with PTA and the presence or absence of memory (Cook, 1972; Mandleberg, 1975; Russell, 1971); with performance on the Wechsler Memory Scale (Brooks, 1976); or the Wechsler Adult Intelligence Scale (Bond, 1990). Likewise, the Glasgow Coma Scale has been used as comparison to behavioral problems post-morbidly (Levin, Benton & Grossman, 1983); to speed of recovery (Zwaagstra, Schmidt, and Vanier, 1996). Pharmacologic interventions for agitation post-morbid have been analyzed (Fugate et.al, 1997a). Length of time post-injury and degree of emotional stress exhibited on standard tests such as the Katz Adjustment Scale and the Minnesota Multiphasic Personality Inventory (MMPI) have been analyzed (Fordyce, Roueche, & Prigatano, 1983).

As noted by Prigatano (1986), the scientific investigations are necessary but are not sufficient. Individuals with TBI have a personal reaction to their deficits. These reactions present a sequelae all their own and are influenced by the premorbid intellectual and sociocultural characteristics of the individual. The interaction of the brain injury and the individual him/herself produces a complex symptom picture often involving personality disorders, such as emotions, motivation, and cognitive functioning (Prigatano, 1986). The importance of the individual's personality variables for rehabilitation outcome introduced another wave of TBI rehabilitation literature, yet still neglected to operatively define motivation (Levin, Benton, & Grossman, 1983; Prigatano, 1989b; Valenstein & Heilman, 1979).

Rehabilitation Program Trends

With the exponential growth of rehabilitation facilities specializing in the care of the traumatically brain injured individual, so followed the plethora of literature debating treatment styles for their outcome effectiveness (Ellerd, Moore, Speer, & Lackey, 1994; Kreutzer, Gordan & Wehman, 1989; Leland, Lewis, Hinman, & Carrillo, 1988; Prigatano, 1989a). Characteristics of behavior were discussed and cautions were made for therapists, "the unsophisticated therapist will often assume at this point [patient non-compliant with daily schedule due to memory, planning, organizational deficits] that the patient is just 'unmotivated' " (Prigatano, 1989, p. 140).

The return to "productive activity," "empowering the individual with a disability," "social reintegration" all have been featured in the literature

30

(Cicerone, 1989; Crisp, 1994; Olney and Salomone, 1992). The literature on rehabilitation programs and vocational/social reintegration generally tends to focus upon the individual's access to rehabilitative services, personality/behavioral deficits, cognitive problems, and social skills. Variations of the same theme of individualized client service plans (CSP) as identified by Haffey and Lewis (1989) are plentiful in the literature. The following excerpt from Haffey and Lewis (1989) is illustrative of many entries:

> The novel feature of this CSP is that projected outcome goals are specified, essential events in the client and environment are identified, and classes of disability or impairment are rated according to the degree to which they currently pose a barrier to outcome goal attainment....The intended result of this CSP process is better targeting of rehabilitative services. This is the first step to improve rehabilitative effectiveness and efficiency. The second is structuring rehabilitative interventions to promote optimal levels of skills mastery, generalization, and maintenance.... This practice is especially important when treating TBI persons with motivational or denial problems. If these clients do not believe program objectives are relevant, they will likely be resistant to treatment. (p. 151-154)

As noted in the above excerpt, "[t] his practice [structuring] is especially important when treating TBI persons with motivational or denial problems." Many similar studies have a similar "motivational" weakness to report. That is, the study shows the importance of some rehabilitative technique, especially in light of the "unmotivated patient" – but how does one motivate him/her? The question continues to beg for an answer in the literature.

Family Matters

Certainly not to be overlooked are the wealth of studies on the effects of traumatic brain injury and the family members of the survivor (Fugate et. al,

31

1997a; Rape, Bush, & Slavin, 1992; Willer, Allen, Liss, & Zicht, 1991).

Problems associated with a disability from TBI such as interpersonal problems, aggressiveness or social inappropriateness, depression, and cognitive impairments especially memory and communicative skills were among some of the areas of investigations in like studies. Most times, motivational difficulties were mentioned, but no offerings were made for overcoming these difficulties on a day-to-day basis.

Self-Awareness

The uniqueness of an individual, that is who he/she believes he/she is, how he/she presumes he/she is perceived, how he/she behaves, is damaged when one suffers a traumatic brain injury. Many studies have been conducted studying the survivors' self-concept and self-awareness (Chittum, Johnson, Chittum, Guericio & McMorrow, 1996; Fleming, Strong & Ashton, 1996; Klonoff, O'Brien, Prigatano, Chiapello, & Cunningham, 1989; Vanderhaeghen, 1985). One of the most confirming studies for this study was that of Nochi, "Loss of Self," (1997). In his qualitative study, Nochi found that individuals with TBI experience a loss of self in several ways although they may successfully avoid or minimize the loss through compensatory strategies. Nochi (1997) found that individuals with (1) "TBI find it difficult to develop clear self-knowledge," (2) "loss of self is conspicuous when they compare their present status with their past in many aspects of their lives," and (3) "their senses of self are threatened by labels that they feel society imposes upon them." Although his work was masterful, its scope did not include any study of motivational strategies an individual with TBI might use to overcome some or all of his/her loss of self. The question remains unanswered.

Medical Jurisprudence

As noted in the overview of this section, the specialty of traumatic brain injury rehabilitation grew from the mounting costs of post-injury care. The financial burden not only to the families of survivors but also to the community continues to spiral. Medical, rehabilitative, and insurance costs are not the only escalating concerns. The litigation now involved demands that the legal profession is cognizant of the potential deficits from traumatic brain injury (Abrams and Twiggs, 1995; Bee, 1994; Cahn, 1996; Davis, 1990; Nemeth, 1988; Simkins, 1994; Stern, 1996). While this study is certainly not a legal one, the sense of importance given to motivation post-injury for the TBI survivor is well illustrated in this legal entry from Cahn, (1997):

> Such patients [TBI] may look depressed and without motivation and drive, (Duffy & Campbell, 1994) with an indifference to circumstances....Loss of motivation, which, as noted above, may look like depression, is a serious problem in TBI patients (Prigatano, 1986; Duffy & Campbell, 1994; Mega & Cummings, 1994). It is, however, not always related to depression. Such patients may insist that they want to accomplish a task and that they are not trying to procrastinate or be lazy; consequently, depression may not be involved. Yet these patients are unable to accomplish much either at work or home. This loss of drive is due to problems with impaired executive functions (which involve skills such as initiation, persistence, organization, and planning, to be discussed later in this article.)
>
> ...Decreased motivation can have a profound effect on a person's life (Lezak, 1995). In simple terms, all the plans, good intentions, intelligence, and skills are worthless if they cannot be implemented. The ability to 'get

into gear' and actually do something is of paramount importance to successful functioning on a daily basis. (p. 30)

Motivation is certainly recognized as important, but to date there appear to be no guidelines on materializing it for rehabilitation purposes. How does the rehabilitation specialist encourage the individual with a brain injury to be motivated to improve? What are the signs of "a motivated client"? What are the triggers for motivation? What is motivation for the individual with TBI? None of these questions have been addressed in the traumatic brain injury literature reviewed nor did they surface in global computer searches. Finding no answers in the traumatic brain injury rehabilitation literature, I turned to the general patient education literature focusing upon health models and most closely aligned to motivational concerns, that of compliance.

Health Models

Health care workers involved at every level of care from entry emergency treatment to acute bedside attendance to restorative guidance all seek to assist the patient in achieving self-management of his/her medical condition. Patient self-management, often viewed as synonymous with compliance, is a popular topic in health care research.

Three of the most popular models commonly used in self-management education have been the Health Belief Model, the PRECEDE Model, and recently, the Transtheoretical Model.

The Health Belief Model

The Health Belief Model is one of the oldest and most widely used models. The model was created during the 1950's by a group of social psychologists at the U.S. Public Health Service to predict health behaviors, specifically to explain why people did not go for tuberculosis screenings. Originally, the model was based upon the work of social psychologist Kurt Lewin. The model provides a tool for understanding the patient's perception of disease and his decision-making process in the consumption of health care services. Over the years the model has been adapted to consider the consumption of health care services in the presence of chronic illness (Janz and Becker, 1984) or in situations where health promotion is desirable (Pender, 1975). Educators such as Rankin and Stallings (1996) note that the model is often used in patient education research for compliance prediction as well as a tool for gaining a better understanding of the patient's motivation for seeking and obtaining services. The basis of the Health Belief Model is that people act on the basis of perceptions. The model can be divided into two categories, perceived threat and expectations. According to the model, the patient will seek health care if he/she: 1) Perceives that he/she has a disease or condition or is likely to contract it. 2) Perceives that the disease or condition is harmful and has serious consequences. 3) Believes that the suggested health intervention is of value. 4) Believes that the effectiveness of the treatment is worth the cost and barriers he/she must confront.

The PRECEDE Model

The PRECEDE Model (**P**receding, **R**einforcing, **E**nabling **C**auses in **E**ducational **D**iagnosis and **E**valuation) suggests looking at three factors when planning educational programs for patients: predisposing, enabling, and reinforcing factors. The health educator is encouraged by this model to look for the predisposing factors of the patient, that is, the beliefs and benefits of the illness or injury. The educator is guided by this model to seek the enabling factors such as resources and skills mastery for each patient. The major objective in the enabling stage is to give the patient control over his/her life. Finally once a patient has elected to do something, reinforcing is needed to encourage maintenance.

While both of these models are based upon the individual's beliefs changing behavior, the dominant focus of the medical approach to the study of self-management has been to seek explanations in terms of treatment, for example, the nature of the drug and the complexity of the treatment regime (Haynes et. al, 1979).

Transtheoretical Model

Recently in the medical literature, there have been advancements in attempts to understand human motivation in health promotion. Prochaska has developed a model of health behavior (Prochaska et. al, 1994) that he calls a transtheoretical model. (Table 1) This model is an attempt to explain why some people do not modify risky behaviors despite having the relevant information to do so. Prochaska and his colleagues have constructed this model in light of

36

addictive behaviors, such as diet, weight control, smoking cessation, and sexual behavior as related to HIV infection (Prochaska, Redding, Harlow, Rossi & Velicer, 1994). Prochaska and his colleagues proposed that the stages of change are a "developmental sequence of motivational readiness" that include precontemplation, contemplation, preparation, action, and maintenance (Prochaska, et. al, 1994, p. 473). They noted that the stages are not linear and that a patient may cycle in and out of each level multiple times.

Table 1. Prochaska's Transtheoretical Model of Motivation and Change

Stage of Change	Period of Time/Characteristics	Intervention
Precontemplation	• 6 months	Consciousness raising
	•Very little intent to change	
	• Resistant to change- defensive	
Contemplation	• Variable, usually 6 months— years	Self-reevaluation
	• More serious about changing	
	• Ambivalent about costs and benefits	
Preparation	• Variable period of time	Self-liberation
	• Preliminary attempts at healthy behavior	
Action	• Usually lasts up to 6 months	Helping relationships
	• Efforts interspersed with recidivism and relapse	
Maintenance	• Begins 6 months after successful behavior change in the action stage; may last	Stimulus control
	• Relapse may occur but less likely	

The value of this model is its potential to predict the 'teachable moment.' Prochaska, et. al, suggested that interventions to motivate people need to be tailored for each stage.

Compliance

Recently in the nursing literature, the term compliance itself has been critiqued and other terms such as empowerment, partnership, reciprocity have surfaced as the focus of patient education (Falvo, 1994). Physicians consider the motivated patient one who follows his/her orders exactly; for the nurse or rehabilitation worker, the motivated patient begins to engage in self-management; and for the health psychologists the motivated patient has knowledge of his/her illness or disability (Falvo, 1994; Rankin and Stallings, 1996). While each of these three groups approach the study of self-management in a different manner, they each use a common word in speaking of the requirement to achieve effective patient education: motivation.

A first challenge for the health care worker is to understand motivation itself, and its relationship to patient knowledge and action, then harness it for the good of the patient. Understanding a patient's motivation is not like reading a dial; a patient's life cannot be separated from his or her context. Therefore, in addition to the individual characteristics that define the patient (illness, perceptions, prognosis, demographics), aspects of the individual as a member of a group of significant others (health care workers, family, friends) whose beliefs, words, and actions contribute to the motivation toward health must be considered (Babcock and Miller, 1994; Loring, 1996; Redman, 1993). In defining patient education (rehabilitation), it is easy to understand the common link between self-management and motivation:

> Patient education is the process of *influencing behavior*, producing changes in knowledge, attitudes, and skills required to maintain and improve health. The process may begin with the imparting of information,

but it also includes interpretation and integration of information in such a manner as to bring about attitudinal or *behavioral changes* that benefit a person's health status. [italics mine] (Simonds, 1979)

Because patient education/rehabilitation to achieve self-management is a process, it occurs over a period of time and requires an ongoing assessment of the patient's knowledge, attitudes, skills, and actions.

> The motivational level of the client with brain injury and family is crucial to the rehabilitation outcome. Unfortunately, many clients and their families are told soon after the client sustains traumatic head injury that the prognosis for recovery is poor and most recovery will occur within the first six months with very little recovery after the first year. Thomsen (1981) reported that significant cognitive changes can take place many years after severe head trauma. Motivation can be viewed as having four components: 1) hope, 2) patience, 3) effort, and 4) trust. Hope is the main catalyst for creating high levels of motivation. Clients quickly become impatient and try to speed up the recovery process by engaging in activities (e.g., going back to work, driving a car) for which they are not ready. As a result, they frequently encounter failure. This should be avoided since it undermines motivation. Clients and their family are quick to verbalize a wish to participate in the rehabilitation program, but effort may ebb if clients or family fear that their effort will not help. The rehabilitation plan must have the trust and support of the client and family before they will be motivated to participate in it. (Ostwald, 1989, p.24)

Unfortunately, the above entry is one of the longer discussions of motivation in the literature. The four components mentioned, hope, patience, effort and trust, are the closest I found in the literature to actual directional research on the "how" of motivation. I offer two other examples; both fall short of any directives:

Example 1:

> They [rehabilitation and behavioral management] provide structure, timely and appropriate reinforcement, motivation, and explanations of patients' functioning…. However, denial has adaptive bases as well, primarily the prevention of a catastrophic reaction. The more awareness a patient has, the more likely depression will affect motivation and self-belief.

40

Paradoxically, denial helps maintain emotional stability and motivation. (Armstrong, 1991, p. 21)

Example 2:

Motivation and attitude are two major factors which most frequently affect a client's entry into the vocational rehabilitation process. Unresolved issues relative to adjustment to disability can work together with problems in motivation and attitude as significant barriers to vocational rehabilitation success. (Ninomiya, et.al, in Ashley, and Krych, 1995, p. 375)

My search of the general patient education literature reflecting upon motivational characteristics of patients revealed no single common factor that caused a patient to be "unmotivated" or "motivated" for that matter. Rather, the motivated patients all seemed to be triggered by different things, individualized likes and dislikes (Cameron & Best, 1987; Cramer, 1991a; Cramer, 1991b; Davies, 1979; Damrosch, 1991; Green, 1987; Haynes, Sackett, &Taylor, 1979; Irwin, et. al, 1993; Jenny, 1983; Mullinax, 1995; Owens, Larrat & Fretwell, 1991; Ross, 1991; Roth, 1987; Slifer, et. al, 1993; Smith et. al, 1987; Spilker, 1991; Tickle-Degnen & Rosenthal, 1992; Wuest, 1993). The individual's readiness or motivation to change the reasons one wants to change and the obstacles encountered in change are important factors to be considered, but there were no specific tips on "how" to assist the patient/client in achieving these goals motivationally.

Since there were no formidable motivation discussions found in the TBI rehabilitation or patient education literature, I sought to integrate the literature of classroom and educational psychology motivational research. Motivational studies in these fields are plentiful; however only the theories I felt most closely related to unlocking the motivational secrets of the TBI population are discussed.

41

Motivation to Change

Although it is common to measure motivation in terms of behavior, there is not one feature or characteristic of behavior that defines motivation. In fact, there is little agreement among researchers regarding a single definition of motivation, probably because the definition of motivated behavior is more dependent upon theoretical commitments of the researcher than upon any specific behavior. Motivation seems to be neither a fact of experience nor a fact of behavior, but more an idea of a concept introduced when we try to explain behavior (Bolles, 1975).

Motivation

…is the concept used when we describe the forces acting on or within an organism to initiate and direct behavior. We also use the concept of motivation to explain the differences in the intensity of behavior. More intense behaviors are considered to be the result of higher levels of motivation. Additionally, we often use the concept of motivation to indicate direction of behavior. (Petri,1991, p. 3)

In the patient educational situation, motivation addresses the willingness of the patient to put effort into learning and to follow medical regime, either advice or treatment. Motivation is not a unitary concept variable only by intensity or amount as many believe. Often the action appears the same from one individual to another yet the motivation for the action is different (Reeve, 1996).

The purpose of this study is to develop a theory of motivation, therefore, there is no atheoretical definition available. The picture of motivation, then, is grounded in a framework of various motivational theories. Motivation to change will be discussed in light of the three major divisions of theories of motivational drives that most closely influence the rehabilitation efforts for the individual with a traumatic brain injury: extrinsic, expectancy-value, and needs based.

EXTRINSIC THEORY OF MOTIVATION

External contingencies are the defining qualities of extrinsic motivation. "Extrinsic motivation is a means-to-an-end type of motivation in which the means is the behavior and the end is some attractive consequence or prevention of an unattractive consequence" (Reeve, 1996, p. 6). While extrinsic and intrinsic (internal) motivation can appear the same outwardly, the defining difference is the source of energy for the action. For extrinsic motivation, the power is environmental, that is, from outer sources while the intrinsically motivated individual is energized from within. Research has shown that extrinsic rewards and/or constraints can decrease intrinsic motivation (Deci & Ryan, 1985, Lepper & Greene, 1978). In the well-known research of Lepper, Greene and Nisbett, (1973), in which they experimented with preschool children drawing a picture for extrinsic rewards, three phenomena were noted: (1) both intrinsic and extrinsic motivation do exist, (2) rewarding children and monitoring their task engagement can have detrimental effects on intrinsic motivation, and (3) the anticipation of the reward itself is the undermining effect for intrinsic motivation.

The study of extrinsic motivation, of course, has as its beginnings, the behavioral experiments with laboratory animals' response to stimulus. Rehabilitation techniques employed for individuals with TBI are often extrinsic in nature and thus do not necessarily foster self-awareness, which should be the one of the goals of rehabilitation (Prigatano, 1986). While extrinsic motivational techniques may be an excellent way to entice the individual with a TBI in the early stages of recovery, it is imperative that he/she is ultimately progressing in his/her rehabilitation efforts with some strength of intrinsic drive so that when the extrinsic reward is no longer available, the inner drive is still present to command the individual's involvement in his/her program.

EXPECTANCY-VALUE VIEWS OF MOTIVATION

Motivation driven by the Atkinson expectancy-value theory (1964) involves many emotions. According to Atkinson, the individual must not only expect to succeed at a task, but also must see personal value of some sort attached to the successful completion of the task. The expectancy-value for the patient is often spoken of in the medical literature. For example Damrosch, (1991) stated that "[i]n terms of motivating health behavior change, the research findings indicate the importance of the client's belief in the severity of the threat to health and personal vulnerability, as well as in the feasibility and effectiveness of a particular health measure" (p. 842).

For the TBI population, I see three key concepts embedded in the expectancy-value theory: self-efficacy and volition.

Self-Efficacy

Bandura cited (1982) the importance of self-efficacy in health-related activities such as controlling tension headaches, pain management, smoking cessation, and cardiac rehabilitation. Bandura challenged health professionals to conduct "self-efficacy probes during the course of treatment [to] provide helpful guides for implementing a program of personal change" (1998). The simple definition offered by Bandura for self-efficacy is "a judgment of one's capability to accomplish a certain level of performance" (1998). According to Bandura (1986):

> 1) the state of belief in one's ability is a good predictor or motivation and 2) In addition one's self-efficacy beliefs can be enhanced through performance mastery, modeling, reinterpretation of physiological symptoms and social persuasion. 3) Finally, enhanced self-efficacy leads to improved behaviors, motivation, thinking patterns and emotional well being. It is not concerned with the skills one has but with judgments of what one can do with whatever skills one possesses. (1998)

Citing research studies with patients recovering from myocardial infarction (MI) (1986), Bandura noted that there are four sources for a patient to measure his/her self-efficacy: (1) performance attainment, as shown in mastery by the patient, (2) vicarious experience, as in visualizing others being successful and imaging self in that position, (3) verbal persuasion, as in the supportive talk others provide to help the individual into believing in self, and (4) physiological states, as internal cues such as arousal.

Self-efficacy is situation-specific. Self-efficacy deals with one's perception or belief that he/she can accomplish some particular future behavior. In this way, it is predictive. One's efficacy for future performance is a good predictor of actual future health performance (Loring, 1996). For the TBI

45

population, being successful in regaining each part of personal functionality,

whether it be cognitive or physical, is a constant self-efficacy testing ground.

Volition

Occupational therapy has observed the value of understanding patients'

meaning and volition for life through individuals' personal narratives for over four

decades (Bateson, 1956; Engelhardt, 1977; Gergen & Gergen, 1988; Helfrich &

Kielhofner, 1993; Yerxa, 1967). A discussion of narratives is beyond the scope

of this study. However, its value to the TBI population is shown in the study of

Helfrich, Kielhofner, and Mattingly. This study argued that

> …persons interpret and anticipate their lives in volitional narratives that
> organize their sense of personal causation, interests, and values into a
> coherent schema. These volitional narratives also relate an array of past,
> present, and potential life events into systematic wholes. Moreover,
> persons remember past experiences and anticipate an imagined future from
> the perspective of these narratives. The concept of volitional narratives
> builds the interdisciplinary argument that persons organize their self
> knowledge and choices through narratives, that is, stories they tell
> themselves and others (1994).

Corno (1993) explained that colloquially, volition, is taken to mean

"strength of will." This expression, continued Corno, suggests a continuum with

weakness as its opposite. Volition is also associated with a variety of

characteristics attributed to individuals who apply themselves diligently to any

task they undertake. Corno spoke of a "crossing the Rubicon" effect in which an

initial forcing of oneself eventually precipitates a more effortless engagement with

a task. Involvement is the consequence or possible outcome of volition according

to Corno. As explained by Corno, "the primary role of volition is in the

46

management and implementation of goals. Motivational factors, in contrast, help to determine goals" (1993, p. 17). Corno noted in her explanation of "Crossing the Rubicon" that

> much is assumed to depend on the cognitive-intellectual aptitude, as well as individual reinforcement history and context …research that includes volitional processes in the same equation with motivation and cognition can be use to illustrate how these relations may be mediated by a number of task and individual difference factors, of which volition is but one (1993, p. 18).

NEEDS-BASED VIEWS OF MOTIVATION

A third approach to motivation is represented by theories that describe motivation as deriving from basic human needs such as competence, affiliation, and autonomy. Here, I discuss four different lines of work that are based on this approach and that I see as relevant to my study.

Self-determination Theory

Deci and Ryan made an important additional distinction in behaviors that are intentional or motivated (Deci, et. al, 1991). They distinguished between self-determined and controlled types of intentional regulation. "Motivated actions are self-determined to the extent that they are engaged in wholly volitionally and endorsed by one's sense of self, whereas actions are controlled if they are compelled by some interpersonal or intrapsychic force. When a behavior is self-determined, the regulatory process is choice, but when it is controlled, the regulatory process is compliance (or in some cases defiance)" (Deci, et. al, p. 326-327). Self- determination theory presents postulates about basic psychological needs that are inherent in life: the needs for competence, relatedness, and autonomy. According to Deci and Ryan, competence involves understanding how to attain external and internal outcomes; relatedness has to do with developing secure and satisfying connections with others in social circles, and autonomy represents the self-initiating and self-regulating of one's own activities. The significance of this theory for the TBI population is that it would support approaches in which clients are encouraged to accept responsibility for their behavior, so their rehabilitation efforts will persist in the absence of the rehabilitation setting or rewards. Furthermore, when a TBI client feels that he/she is in control of his/her life, the person's motivation energy seems to be greater.

Flow/Involvement

Csikszentmihalyi reminded us that 2300 years ago Aristotle concluded that more than anything else, men and women seek happiness in life. We seek everything else, such as health, beauty, money, power, possessions, because we think they will make us happy. After decades of studying people, Csikszentmihalyi discovered that happiness is not something that happens.

> It is not the result of good fortune or random chance. It is not something money can buy or power command. It does not depend upon outside events, but, rather, on how we interpret them. Happiness, in fact, is a condition that must be prepared for, cultivated, and defended privately by each person. People who learn to control inner experience will be able to determine the quality of their lives, which is as close as any of us can come to being happy (1990, p. 2).

Because perceptions are most often molded by forces outside one's control, it is not surprising that people generally believe others determine their fate or happiness. However, as Csikszentmihalyi explained, there are times when one feels in control of his/her actions, masters of one's own fate. When that feeling occurs, the individual experiences an exhilaration, an internal synergy, for which he/she has longed. This feeling, Csikszentmihalyi labeled *optimal experience*. An optimal experience, according to Csikszentmihalyi, is an occasion when an individual becomes so engrossed by the activity undertaken that he/she loses himself/herself in the task and nothing else matters; the experience itself is so enjoyable that people will do it even at great cost. According to Csikszentmihalyi (1990), what leads to this sense of an optimal experience

> is order in consciousness...when psychic energy—or attention—is invested in realistic goals, and when skills match the opportunities for action. The pursuit of a goal brings order in awareness because a person must concentrate attention on the task at hand and momentarily forget everything else. (p.6)

During times of optimal experience, the individual experiences all the positive aspects of the human experience—joy, creativity, a total involvement with life. Csikszentmihalyi called such a feeling *flow*. Csikszentmihalyi (1990) described flow as a process of achieving happiness by gaining control over one's own inner consciousness. This control might be achieved most easily when tasks are intrinsically rewarding. Every flow activity examined by Csikszentmihalyi , whether competition, chance, or other experiences, had this is common: "It [the activity] provided a sense of discovery, a creative feeling of transporting the person to a new reality. It pushed the person to higher levels of performance, and led to previously undreamed-of states of consciousness. In short, it transformed the self by making it more complex" (1990, p. 74).

Figure 2.1 illustrates Csikszentmihalyi's theory of flow activity for an individual with a TBI. Let us assume that the figure represents a specific rehabilitation activity—relearning the sequence for a shower. The two theoretically most important dimensions of the experience, according to Csikszentmihalyi, are challenges and skills. They are represented on the two axes of the diagram. The letter A represents Myrtle, a young lady recovering from a TBI. The diagram shows Myrtle at four different times. When she first starts attempting to recall how to shower, she cannot remember to take her clothes off, nor any of the following steps we all take for granted daily. Myrtle has practically no skills, and the only challenge she faces is remembering to take off her clothes first, A1. While this is not a very difficult task, Myrtle is likely to enjoy it right now for her skills are so rudimentary at this time in recovery. Therefore, for the current time, Myrtle is in flow simply by enjoying the fact that she has recalled this first step. However, with repeated practice day after day, Myrtle will soon learn these steps and will become bored just recalling the sequence to take off her clothes, A2. At this point, Myrtle realizes that she feels embarrassed to stand naked with the rehabilitation worker day after day not knowing what to do next, yet realizing that she cannot rejoin the group's activities until she is clean and clothed. This makes her feel anxious, A3. Neither boredom (A2) nor anxiety (A3) are positive experiences; neither create that feeling of an optimal experience. Therefore, Myrtle's only choice is to return to her flow state by increasing the challenges, learning now how actually to shower. With this recognition and

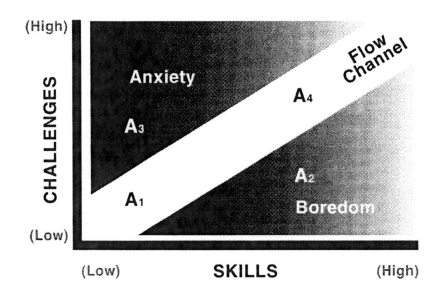

33333Figure 2.1.   Csikszentmihalyi's theory of flow.

51

pursuit, Myrtle becomes A4. Of course, she can drop out all together and either adopt another goal or go into depression. Her other option would be to return to A1, a lesser task. A1 and A4 both represent situations in which Myrtle was in flow. Although theoretically both are enjoyable, they are different in that A4 is a more complex experience than A1 because it involves greater challenges and demands more skills. The motivation to enjoy success will only be stable as she moves up the ladder of challenges and skills. Once a goal has been obtained, no matter how small, it is difficult to remain in the stream of flow for long because the individual falls to the side in boredom.

In his studies of individuals surviving severe ordeals physically, Csikszentmihalyi discovered that flow is equally viable for them. "Those who know how to transform a hopeless situation into a new flow activity that can be controlled will be able to enjoy themselves, and emerge stronger from the ordeal" (1990, p. 203). The transformation from tragedy to flow is accomplished in three steps, according to Csikszentmihalyi (1990, p. 202-208):

1. Believing that destiny is still in one's own hands or unself-conscious self-assurance. Do not doubt inner resources.

2. Focusing attention on the world, expending energy outside of self.

3. Discovering new solutions, whether direct or indirect. A direct solution is to focus attention upon obstacles to achieving one's goals and then to move them out of the way. The indirect approach is to focus on the entire situation, including self, and discover alternatives.

The control of one's own life leads to flow experiences (Schallert and Reed, 1997). However, at times an individual becomes frustrated when the experiences of life are not salient. How does this feeling affect motivation? Eric Klinger's theory for incentive motivation centers around the basic concept of meaningfulness in life.

Theory of Disengagement

For Klinger (1975), incentives serve as mediators between stimulus and response. That is, individuals pursue objects, events, and experiences that are emotionally important, or meaningful. Klinger made an important differentiation between incentives and goals. Incentives are events or objects that are valued. Goals are objects or events for which individuals are willing to work. An individual may value something and, therefore, have incentive to achieve it; but it may not be a goal, that is the individual may not be willing to work toward achieving the incentive. When the individual decides to pursue an incentive, it becomes a goal. A goal, then, influences behavior, according to Klinger, until the individual either reaches it, or becomes disengaged from it. Klinger postulated that an individual disengages from a goal toward which he/she is working when it becomes unreachable. Klinger offered five stages for disengagement:

1. Invigoration. An individual often pursues a goal more vigorously if it appears to be unreachable. The blocked incentive becomes more attractive for a period of time.
2. Primitivization. If the goal remains unreachable, then behavior can become primitive, even destructive.
3. Aggression. Aggressive behavior often precedes the final efforts of an individual to reach a goal and may be the last step prior to giving up.

4. Depression. Mild disappointment to extreme depression can occur if all attempts to reach the goal fail.

5. Recovery. While there are no real indicators for the triggers of recovery, it usually occurs and the individual pursues another goal.

Klinger's disengagement theory is of value to the TBI population for so many goals an individual may have had prior to his/her injury become unattainable. It is imperative for the individual to establish a new set of reachable goals in order to experience Csikszentmihalyi's flow in life. The individual must learn to recognize the optimal experience which produces flow.

Learning

The individual recovering from a traumatic brain injury is faced with the challenge of relearning previous knowledge and/or skills. The range of knowledge to be regained may be minimal or great, but the needs of a learner and the individual with a TBI are the same. A major function of rehabilitation is to elicit positive behaviors from individuals through education and empower them to control their recovery progress and future. This empowerment is sought through an analysis of the individual's health needs, social needs, personal goals and his/her capacity to learn. Because an individual's life is influenced by his/her environment, an understanding of how that environment effects him/her became an important area for review in this study. Therefore, literature from the field of educational psychology was studied to gain guidelines for the learners from a constructivist viewpoint.

Socioconstructive, Sociocultural Views of Learning

The term socioconstructivist view of learning implies that knowledge is (1) a social product, (2) evolved from negotiation, and (3) influenced by culture and history (Prawat and Floden, 1994). Resnick explained it this way: "...cognition that is not bounded by the individual brain or mind." (1991, p. 1). Resnick continued to explain his phenomenon of shared cognition, "a view that most knowledge is an interpretation of experience, an interpretation based on schemas, often idiosyncratic at least in detail, that both enable and constrain individuals' processes of sense-making" (Resnick, 1991, p. 1) Vygotsky suggested that social experience can shape the kinds of interpretive processes available to individuals (Vygotsky, 1978). The foundation for Vygotsky's analysis of human mental functioning, as noted by Wertsch and Rupert (1993), was his claim that "the social dimension of consciousness is primary in time and in fact. The individual dimension of consciousness is derivative and secondary" (Vygotsky, as cited in Wertsch and Rupert, 1993, p. 227). Vygotsky's belief of human mental functioning motivated his analyses of the internalization of speech, of the "zone of proximal development," and his "general genetic law of cultural development."

> Any function in the child's cultural development appears twice, or on two planes. First it appears on the social plane, and then on the psychological plane. First it appears between people as an *inter*-psychological category, and then within the child as an intrapsychological category, [italics mine]. This is equally true with regard to voluntary attention, logical memory, the formation of concepts, and the development of volition.... It goes without saying that internalization transforms the process itself and changes its structure and functions. Social relations or relations among people genetically underlie all higher functions and their

relationships. (Vygotsky as cited in Wertsch and Rupert, 1993, p. 227-228)

Thus, Vygotsky's central claim was that the system of social relationships in which an individual lives and grows is the key to an understanding of the individual's psychological development. The cultural system itself is the product of generations. Vygotsky believed that one's cultural heritage is most ubiquitously expressed in language. Language mediates all thought (Vygotsky, 1994). The genetic law of cultural development has been used frequently to explain education phenomena. For example Shigaki, (1987), noted that the "[t]ransmission of values to the young is crucial to the survival and maintenance of a culture. While the process varies from culture to culture, language plays a central role in inculcating values in all modern societies" (p. 111). Language provides the conduit for interaction, the foundation for a socioconstructivist point of view.

> Language always happens as text, and not as isolated words and sentences. From an aesthetic, social or educational perspective it is the text which is the significant unit of language. Texts arise in specific social situations and they are constructed with specific purposes by one or more speakers or writers. Meanings find their expression in text—though the meanings are outside the text—and are negotiated (about) in texts, in concrete situations of social exchange." (Kress, 1989, p. 18).

Therefore, in this view, an individual needs to be understood as a social agent located in a network of social relations according to Kress. No man is an island — our social relations within our network shape our minds and our thoughts.

Wells (1987) presented communication as inherently problematic because each individual's ideas arise out of unique, personal experiences. Because no two people have the same set of experiences, they can surely not have identical ideas.

56

Furthermore, people do not share language resources, abilities, or codes. Communication is not a replication of experience, rather a representation of real instances. Wells referred to this as negotiated meaning:

> So, when I try to "convey" my ideas to a listener or a reader, there are many steps at which the sharpness and precision of my personal thoughts and feelings become blurred, as I draw from the mental representation of my experience the salient aspects that I decide to communicate, and then select from my linguistic resources the items of vocabulary and grammatical structure that, in my judgment, will most adequately encode them, and finally articulate them in speech or writing. But, of course, all that is available to the receiver is a stream of sounds, with accompanying gestures and intonation, or a sequence of marks on the page, which, in themselves, have no meaning at all. For receivers to understand my meaning, a related process is required in which they judge to match the decoded sequence of sounds or marks. In other words, as a receiver, one never knows what the sender means — what thoughts he or she is trying to communicate; one only knows what thoughts one would have had in mind if one had spoken or written the same sentences oneself. Seen in this light, it is clear that communication must include *collaboration (italics mine)* (Wells, 1987, p. 5)

It should be noted that there is a divided faction regarding an exacting definition of "negotiated meaning." On the one hand, the definition denotes working toward agreement. On the other hand, reference is made to "skillfully overcoming obstacles" (Prawat and Floden, 1994, p. 40). Socially constructed knowledge is created from a shared rather than an individual experience (Prawat and Floden, 1994). Negotiated meaning and how we negotiate it is the infrastructure for Grice's Cooperative Principle and DeBeaugrande's Seven Standards of Textuality. Grice offered the maxims of Quantity, Quality, Relation, and Manner in his efforts to analyze conversations:

> Our talk exchanges do not normally consist of a succession of disconnected remarks, and would not be rational if they did. They are characteristically, to some degree at least, *cooperative efforts* [italics the

author's]; and each participant recognizes in them, to some extent, a common purpose or set of purposes, or at least a mutually accepted direction. This purpose or direction may be fixed from the start (e.g. by an initial proposal of a question of discussion), or may evolve during the exchange; it may be fairly definite, or it may be so indefinite as they leave very considerable latitude to the participants (as in a casual conversation) (Grice, 1975, p. 45).

While the focus of Grice on the cooperative efforts of conversation, DeBeaugrande focuses on the text itself.

DeBeaugrande noted that how our texts function in human interaction can be defined by seven standards: Cohesion, Coherence, Intentionality, Acceptability, Informativity, Situationality, and Intertextuality. In addition to these constitutive principles that define and create the form of behavior identifiable as textual communicating, DeBeaugrande noted that there are three regulative principles that control rather than define text: efficiency, effectiveness, and appropriateness. These standards of textuality, notes DeBeaugrande, entail factors of cognition, planning, and social environment even to merely distinguish what constitutes a text (DeBeaugrande, 1981). Not only are the cooperative efforts and the text themselves important, but according to Kress even the conversational occasion creates specific genres.

> The conventionalised forms of the occasions lead to conventionalised forms of texts, to specific genres. Genres have specific forms and meanings, deriving from and encoding the functions, purposes and meanings of the social occasions. Genres therefore provide a precise index and catalogue of the relevant social occasions of a community at a given time. A few examples of genre are: interview, essay, conversation, sale, tutorial, sports commentary, seduction, office memo, novel, political speech, editorial, sermon, joke, instruction…. (Kress, 1989, p. 19)

Texts are given form and meaning by discourse and genre. Texts are the product of individual speakers who, as social agents, are "themselves formed in discourses through texts, attempting to make sense of the competing, contradictory demands and claims of differing discourses. The history of each individual traces her or his passage through, and experience of a variety of discourses, not haphazardly encountered, but experienced in the contexts of specific social structures and processes" (Kress, 1989, p. 31). These "social structures and processes" are discourse communities.

A key construct in a socioconstructivist approach is that of "discourse community, by which is meant the shared preferred ways of speaking or writing of a group. Each community judges the quality of ideas in part as a function of the extent to which they are expressed, according to community standards" (Resnick, 1991). Resnick pointed to the phenomenon of code-switching to show that people can belong to multiple communities, each enabling and constraining thought in different ways. Which code an individual uses, or which discourse community he/she chooses, is dependent upon particular cognitive situations and his/her past social experience. Although many linguists have offered definitions of discourse communities, such as Freed and Broadhead (1986), "a community sharing rules for the conduct and interpretation of speech...," it is Kress' definition that best clarifies the subject:

> Discourses are systematically-organized sets of statements which give expression to the meanings and values of an institution. Beyond that, they define, describe and delimit what it is possible to say and not possible to say (and by extension — what it is possible to do or not to do with respect to the area of concern of that institution, whether marginally or centrally. A discourse provides a set of possible statements about a given area, and organizes and gives structure to the manner in which a particular topic, object, process is to be talked about. In that it provides descriptions, rules, permissions and prohibitions of social and individual actions. ... Discourses do not exist in isolation but within a larger system of

59

sometimes opposing, contradictory, contending, or merely different discourses. Given that each discourse tends towards the colonization of larger areas, there are dynamic relations between these which ensure continuous shifts and movement, progression or withdrawal certain areas (Kress, 1989, p. 31).

"Different people in different positions at different moments will live in different realities" (Shotter, 1993, p.17). Shotter continued discussion of a fragmented reality by noting that there is a special knowledge each individual must acquire, "how to be a person of this or that particular kind according to the culture into which one develops as child" (1993, p. 19). This knowledge, proposed Shotter, is the kind of knowledge one has from within a situation, a group, a social institution, or society. How then, does one begin to cope with the intertextual, already formulated knowledge, of a community?

Donald Norman, in The Design of Everyday Things (1988), cautioned the reader that we build models that are essential in helping us understand our experiences. We have a model not only for how things may work with people, but how people may work with things. Our models are based upon prior knowledge, real or imaginary, naive or sophisticated. Prior knowledge is "the sum of what an individual knows" (Schallert, 1991) and is molded and influenced by meanings we negotiate with those in our various discourse communities. Our mental models, then represent our socially constructed knowledge. Social construction of meaning was central to Vygotsky. The construct of "scaffolding" evolved from Vygotsky's stress on social interactions and one's "zone of proximal development," "the distance between the actual developmental level as determined by independent problem solving and the level of potential development as determined through problem solving under adult guidance or in collaboration with capable peers" (Vygotsky, in Meyer, 1993, p. 43).

Scaffolding is a collaborative and non-evaluative interaction; therefore, it may

represent the heart of socially constructed knowledge. Meyer noted that

constructing knowledge is a constructive process for giving personal meaning to

experience. A person's interactions within particular context influence this

construction. Neither meaning nor experience remains stable, but rather they co-

evolve as a natural part of human interaction and development (1993). Socially

constructed knowledge emerges from one's intellectual relationship with the

world. This relationship is fluid and permeable. Perceptions play an integral part

in the central role of cognition. "Society, through its use of language and other

artifacts, shapes the individual's view of reality. Through language, members of a

discourse community learn to 'carve out' the world in similar ways; they develop

similar 'anticipations' about external reality" (Prawat and Floden, 1994, p. 44).

In considering the driving forces of motivation in a patient, one of the

most often overlooked motivating factors is that of the communication channels

available to the patient. There are four major communication relationships in the

health care setting: (1) professional-patient, (2) professional-professional, (3)

professional-family (support structure), and (4) patient-family (support structure)

(Northouse and Northouse, 1992). The flow of communication, whether

excellent, moderate, or weak, will affect the patient's readiness to change.

Communication itself is inherently problematic and thus collaboration is always

required — an attempt by each to understand the intention of the other and to

respond in terms of that understanding (Wells, 1987). For the patient,

communication difficulties can be the source of motivational problems. Which code an individual uses, or which discourse community he/she chooses, is dependent upon the particular cognitive situations and past social experience. Misinterpreted communication in or between any of the four health care relationships can impede the patient's flow activity in self-management.

The medical implication of socially constructed meanings is rather clear. Interaction is constantly being redefined to create social reality. It is a negotiation with an emphasis on interpersonal interaction which acknowledges power. The nurse-patient interaction can be considered an example of this type of relationship. Holmes (1996) found:

> As the interactions between physicians and patients move toward a more facilitative level, as opposed to a one-sided paternalistic level, the process of negotiation assumes more importance. Articulating behaviors on the part of both physicians and patients that contribute to the negotiation of meaning may serve to increase patient understanding and patient satisfaction (p. 176).

Negotiated meaning that produces shared understanding in any of the four relationship groups will contribute to behavior change and maintenance.

Therefore, the way one learns and comprehends is an important element of how TBI survivors can internalize information and seek to reconstruct a new self.

Integrative Summary

Motivation is a complex and multifaceted process. The importance of motivation in the recovery from traumatic brain injury is clear. Previous research in the field of neurology and rehabilitation have recognized the importance of emotions and motivation in the recovery process from brain injury. Studies in

62

these fields have identified some of the problem areas, that is, stumbling blocks for the individual struggling in a recovery program or the outcome of an unmotivated client. However, no solutions have been offered for the triggers of motivation, what it is that does or does not generate energy to accomplish tasks in rehabilitation efforts. Research from the field of education has provided multiple theories regarding motivation in all three major divisions recognized medically: biological, behavioral, cognitive. Likewise, literature from the field of educational research has yielded the tools for understanding how people learn. Applying the classroom motivational and learning findings to traumatic brain injury rehabilitation should provide needed information that will begin to address the motivational patterns that result in increased productivity hence progress for the individual with a TBI. The literature pertinent to the outcomes of this motivation will be addressed in Chapter 6.

CHAPTER 3

PRELIMINARY STUDIES

"Like living, recovery is a never-ending, ongoing process,
it's a case of learning how to live in a different body and brain."
                                    -David, Preliminary Study 1

Overview

To experience the emergence of a theory by studying the phenomenon it represents is much like experimenting with a kaleidoscope. As the image will change with each turn of the wheel or variance of light on the kaleidoscope so did my perception of "motivation" during my initial data collecting from January, 1997 to May, 1997.

In Preliminary Study 1, I sought to identify, if possible, the common motivational feelings among persons with brain injury. What I heard in their comments was the loss of self-identification and their individual struggle to know themselves. Each seemed to struggle with this "new person." As participants reflected upon their struggle to rediscover themselves as persons, they seemed to define their progress in terms of emotions and a time frame. The picture of a timeline of healing began to emerge from the qualitative data, yet was not definable in terms of how it related to the motivational factors I was seeking to identify.

The discovery of "redefining self" as the central phenomenon was the catalyst for Preliminary Study 2 in which I sought to uncover "how" each survivor redefined self. I felt a need to better define "motivation" prior to conducting the main study. During this second study, I discovered that the common interview answers revolved around the "stages" or "phases" or "progression" of recovery. As I progressed in Preliminary Study 2, I returned to the rehabilitation literature and sought a clearer understanding of how a patient "changes" or "progresses" through the "stages" that were being reported to me. The transtheoretical model of health behavior, developed by Prochaska and colleagues (1995) posits that an individual cycles through a "developmental sequence of motivational readiness" any time he/she makes a change in life. My traumatic brain injury (TBI) recovery kaleidoscope began to fall into place after studying the Prochaska model, and listening to many conversations with survivors of traumatic brain injury. Building upon Preliminary Study 1, I was interested in discovering a description of one's progression of recovery in Preliminary Study 2 One participant in Preliminary Study 2, Alicia, explained to me:

> ...it was like I had stages of recovery. At first I was so euphoric when I woke up and realized that I was alive I was just happy to be here and figured I could cope with whatever I'd been left with. But then as I began to get better I wanted my old self back and fought to get there and was angry – that was in like Stage 2. *(sic)* Finally, I decided that I wasn't ever going to be exactly the same but I could be a great person so I had to learn to compensate and get on with life – so I did.

As preparation for the current project discussion, Preliminary Studies 1 and 2 are reviewed.

Preliminary Study 1

The ultimate goal in the rehabilitation of any illness or injury is the return of the patient to his/her ability to function once again as an independent human being. Health care workers involved at every level of care from entry emergency

65

to acute to restorative care all seek to assist the patient in achieving self-management of his/her medical condition. Patient self-management is a popular topic in health care research; however, it is most often discussed in light of "compliance" (Babcock & Miller, 1994; Cramer, 1991a; Cramer & Spilker, 1991; Falvo, 1994; Irwin, Millstein, & Ellen, 1993; Owens, Larrat, & Fretwell, 1991; Rankin & Stallings, 1996; Redman, 1993).

The dominant focus of the medical approach to the study of self-management has been to seek explanations in terms of treatment, as for example, the nature of the drug and the complexity of the treatment regime (Haynes, et.al, 1979). Recently in the nursing literature, the term "compliance" itself has been critiqued and other terms such as "empowerment," "partnership," and " reciprocity" have surfaced as the focus of patient education (Falvo, 1994). Health psychologists approach patient education in terms of the learner, and the knowledge gained. While each of these three groups approach the study of self-management in a different manner, they all use a common word in speaking of a key requirement to achieve effective patient education: motivation.

Statement of Problem/Purpose

My interest was in the interpretation of the term motivation. The patient's readiness or desire to change and the obstacles to change seemed important factors to be considered. Therefore, the purpose for Preliminary Study 1 was to capture the patients' motivational and volitional experiences as they progressed

66

through a rehabilitation program and, from these experiences, attempt to discover the answers to the following research questions:

1. What are the positive and negative factors influencing motivation in the educational practices related to brain injury?

2. Is there a relationship of the comprehension of information regarding brain injury to the volition of self-management?

3. What knowledge is needed by brain injury patients to aid in motivation toward self-management?

Method

Ten participants were identified by asking questions of friends, acquaintances, and by accessing the Internet seeking individuals who had experienced brain injury. In the initial study, no distinction for participant selection was made between acquired (natural causes such as stroke, or tumor) and traumatic (external blow of some sort) injury. The 10 participants ranged in age from 16 to 62 years of age, both men and women. The educational breakdown ranged from high school to post graduate degrees including the Ph.D.

Interviews were conducted with four individuals face-to-face, two individuals via telephone, and four individuals via Internet electronic mail (e-mail). Live interviews were recorded and later transcribed. Online interviews yielded a printout of the computer conversation. The semi-structured interview questions have been included in Appendix B for reference. The data were analyzed first by open coding, that is placing labels on discrete happenings, events, and other instances, then "breaking down, examining, comparing, conceptualizing, and categorizing [the] data" (Strauss & Corbin, 1990, p. 61). The second step of analysis was axial coding, that is "making connections between the categories established in the open coding procedure. According to Strauss and Corbin, this is accomplished by "utilizing a coding paradigm involving conditions, context, action/interactional strategies and consequences" (1990, p. 96). Selective coding completed the analysis process. The process of selective coding is the selection of the core category, systematically relating it to other categories, validating those relationships, and filling in categories that need further refinement and development" (Strauss & Corbin, 1990, p. 116). I discovered that the original research questions I thought keys to understanding rehabilitation efforts of TBI survivors, were in fact, of secondary interest to the participants.

Results

The central phenomenon that emerged was a brain-injured patient's struggle to construct his/her new self. Every brain injured (BI) patient interviewed noted the incredible loss of identity, the loss of the person he/she knew as "self." To protect the identity of participants, all names used in this dissertation are pseudonyms. Self-identity is difficult, as noted by Jim, " …it [traumatic brain injury] is like taking a hammer away from a carpenter and still expecting him to build a house that looks great!" The loss of self and the struggle just to exist while constructing a new self was highlighted in comments by David,

"I can remember the world before and I have not yet let the old David die as I am keeping hope that one day David will return..." Karen also realized that she was a different person, "I want my old body, my old life, back, but since I can't have that, then I know I have to make the best of what I do have. I'm not me anymore." The anguish of the labels placed upon them by society is reflected in the commentary of Joseph, "I gotta act/be like everyone else ...else I'll be considered a "less-than-normal [person]..."

These comments supported the 1997 grounded theory of Nochi in which individuals who had suffered a brain injury (BI) defined "a loss of self." The four types of "loss of self" as named by Nochi are: loss of self-history, the opaque self, the devalued self, and the labeled self (Nochi, 1997). The data gathered in both my preliminary studies confirmed Nochi's findings and while such confirmation was beneficial to my reliability factor in early studies, it still did not answer the question of "what are the triggers of motivation" that energize an individual to work toward recovery.

After sensing the emergence of the theme of loss and struggle to redefine self, I followed-up with the question: "What, in your opinion, has been your greatest struggle in the ordeal?" Perhaps the best summary I can offer for the devastating loss of self and struggle for a new identity that a BI (brain injury) patient experiences is seen in this poem composed by Susan in response to the above question:

> I thought today of who I used to be
> So I looked in the mirror and I saw only me
> I am here, I was, I am just let me be.
> Yes, I am more emotional, Yes, I am angry, Yes, I am sad
> But, I am no less, I just need time to remember and maybe regress,

I must mourn for who I used to be.
Give me time, give me space, don't crowd, don't demand
I will try, I will try, just stand by me.
Give me time, give me space, give me peace and give me air
I still am, I see me, and GOD knows that I try.
Don't expect, don't ask, don't make it too tough
Let me look into the mirror and remember who I am.
Let me cry, let me mourn, let me pour my heart out
I want to scream, I want to shout, for the life that I lost.
I will never be like them, but I can be better
I feel more, I see more, I am what I am.

In the stages of open and axial coding, the above entry is representative of answers I received from interviews with participants, therefore, the category named in the selective stage of coding as the core category was that of reconstruction of self.

Positing the reconstruction of self as the core category, the contextual categories (properties of the main category), seemed to fall into two well-defined large groups. The contextual categories named were: (1) rehabilitation processes including the networking of problems, concerns, and support systems and (2) a factor of time post-injury and the emotional struggles of the recovering brain injury patient. The effectiveness of the interaction of these two groups of variables ultimately defines the consequence category (the outcome), reentry into society for the brain injured person.

Just as there are no two identical brain injuries, there seemed to be no identical path for individual experiences along the rehabilitation pathway. While there are no two identical brain injuries, there are common areas of the brain that can sustain damage, such as the frontal lobe, temporal lobe, occipital lobe, or parietal lobe whose functions are common from one individual to the next. For example, the occipital lobe controls sight in all individuals, but an injury to an individual's occipital lobe does not necessarily mean that he/she will sustain the identical injury as another individual with an occipital lobe injury. Like the similarities of the functionality of the parts of the brain, there seemed to be a similarity to the pattern of growth and maturity through rehabilitation. The grounded theory model that evolved from Preliminary Study 1 is shown in Figure 3.1.

Fortunately for hundreds of thousands of acquired brain injury/traumatic brain injury (ABI/TBI) survivors, there comes the day when they can reenter society as independent, productive persons. They may not be the same persons they were before their illness or injury, but nonetheless they are valuable members of society. Reentry is not an easy undertaking, and it is a process that seems to be done best in gradual steps with patience for the length of time required. Among the ABI/TBI survivors who participated in Preliminary Study 1, none showed obvious physical signs of disability and yet all were still recovering even when 20+ years post-injury. Nevertheless, it was interesting to note the incredible need to reenter society expressed by all, and definite signs of success were exhibited by many.

In Preliminary Study 1, the signs of successful reentry showed this pattern of common experiences:

(1) Most of the participants interviewed (5 of 8) attempted to do community volunteer work prior to entering the paid work force.

> ... A couple of months ago, I rejoined the volunteer program at the hospital where I did my rehab and [I] suggested that we create a program for patients and families to introduce them to the resources for support and information on brain injury available via the internet.
>
> -Ray, online

71

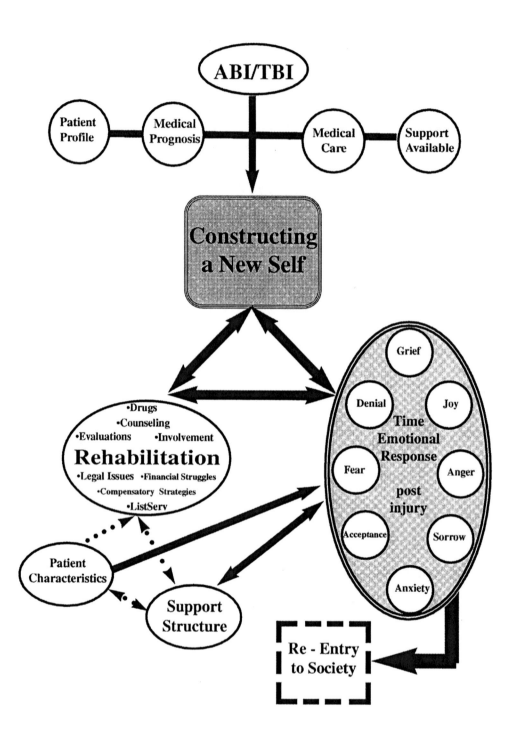

Figure 3.1.   Constructing a new self: A grounded theory model.

I finally backed off and let him be, and he eventually started volunteering at the local police station.

-Elsie, online

(2) Most (6 of 8) struggled, often losing, their first reentry employment

and through the experiences gained valuable personal strategies.

> Set your goals, and if you don't make them today, don't be so hard on yourself, start again tomorrow, and then the next day …you have to give yourself a break sometimes...because its easier to keep trying than to be defeated. Nobody gets only one chance. So keep plugging along. Life is growth. If we were all born knowing everything, life might be a little boring.

-Belinda, interview

> Try this, wake up slowly, never wake up and get up immediately.

-Susan, online

> If worrying about everything is too much, then write it down. Take care of two things a day. Scratch them off. Tell people "NO". Listen to yourself. Your self-esteem should grow.

-Kelly, online

(3) All participants (8 of 8) struggled with reading social cues.

> I also know I had to relearn how to read so-called "social cues" or body language—things like if the person or group I was interacting with was bored, or annoyed, or engaged, whatever. It's like I was so focused on finding words or trying to communicate "outward" that I didn't "get" the subtleties that were being sent out from others. A simultaneous processing issue, too, perhaps.

-Kathleen, online

(4) It was interesting to note that ABI/TBI survivors work through many

problems and rediscover self largely through writing.

> My [written by Bill] Story. A great therapy. When I was in the hospital I was encouraged to write. I wrote letters to the management of the hospital telling them how they needed to run the hospital. Wrote making complaints about different nurses who were treating me as though I was

mentally deranged and completely stupid. I also wrote about my accident, about 20 A4 pages! I've worked on it for 5 years and have said the same thing in one page!!

-Bill, online

I know what you mean about the writing, it does help to share it.

-Kathleen, online

(5) And, most (7 of 8) sensed a deepening faith and religious strength, often writing songs or poems, entered in Appendix C, with religious overtones.

I decided to finally let go of worry and fear and I now go to church and follow the principles of the Bible.

-Ray, online

I think you are on the right track, let go and let God. Do you think there is any truth to "Seek ye first the kingdom of God and His righteousness" and all the rest will fall into place? As a three time brain tumor survivor, I can tell you THERE IS.

-Jeff, online

Discussion

...my feeling is that it is also true that a person with brain injury can have many things—more than one might imagine—if/when you can put your mind to outsmarting the injury rather than either denying it, wishing it would go away or trying to "outmuscle" it.

-Sharon, interview

The thread that seemed to bind every interview together was the patient's desire to regain a sense of self and self worth. The ABI/TBI survivor has had portions of identity snatched from his/her fingertips in a split second. As no two injuries are the same, no two recovery stories are the same; however, three truths were garnered from this study: (1) recovery takes time, (2) the survivor seeks to regain his/her identity and "being-ness," and (3) support teams make the difference. Where is the key, then, to assisting more ABI/TBI survivors to their society reentry debut? From Preliminary Study 1, I was beginning to sense that a progression of recovery, perhaps, was instrumental in the motivational factors. Therefore, preparation was made for Preliminary Study 2 to seek answers to the properties of recovery progress.

Preliminary Study 2

The identification of the brain injured patient's overwhelming need for rediscovery of self and the value of time in recovery were the two compelling ideas I carried away from Preliminary Study 1. I embarked upon Preliminary Study 2 in search of additional insight to these two ideas.

Statement of Problem/Purpose

Preliminary Study 2 was designed with the hopes of answering two research questions:

1. What are the stages of recovery for the brain injured patient?
2. Can technology boost a patient's motivation in any stage?

Drawing upon the interdisciplinary nature of the literature previously reviewed, I focused upon the literature relating specifically to changes or stages in motivation as well as studies addressing the volition of an individual, that is, what moved the motivated individual to action. Recently in the medical literature, advancements in attempts to understand human motivation have been made. As

75

mentioned earlier, Prochaska's transtheoretical model of health behavior (1994) is an attempt to explain why some people do not modify behaviors despite having the relevant information to do so. Prochaska et. al noted that the stages of recovery are not linear and that a patient may cycle in and out of each level multiple times. Prochaska recommended these stages as guidance for tailoring motivation interventions at each stage of change. While Prochaska's model was of a global, clinical nature, I was hopeful that it could offer some guidance for defining "stages" or "progression" of recovery. The studies conducted by Prochaska and colleagues have been conducted with patients who have a *choice* to change, as for example, smokers seeking to quit smoking (Prochaska, DiClemente, Velicer, Ginpil, & Norcross, 1985; Prochaska, Velicer, DiClemente, & Fava, 1988, Prochaska & DiClemente, 1983, 1984; Prochaska, DiClemente, Velicer & Rossi, 1993), or individuals attempting to lose weight (Prochaska & DiClemente, 1985; Prochaska, Norcross, Fowler, Follick, Abrams, 1992), or individuals needing to practice safe sex (Prochaska, Redding, Harlow, Rossi, & Velicer, 1994). This was a major difference in our study population, for my participants did not have a choice but rather were forced into the role of needing to change. Nevertheless, I saw in Prochaska's model a framework for my opening interview questions. Based upon the ideas of Prochaska, I asked each patient if he/she could label his/her progress in the form of a timeline.

Realizing that there had to be "something" that triggered emotions and motivation to action, I reviewed the literature on volition. Lyn Corno (1993) explained that colloquially, volition, is taken to mean "strength of will." This expression, continued Corno, suggests a continuum with weakness as its opposite, as discussed in Chapter 2. Volition is also associated with a variety of characteristics attributed to individuals who apply themselves diligently to any task they undertake. Corno spoke of a "crossing the Rubicon" effect where an initial forcing of oneself eventually precipitates a more effortless engagement with a task. Involvement is the consequence or possible outcome of volition according to Corno.

Method

Preliminary Study 2 was designed around three major activities:

1. I attended the annual Brain Injury Reunion of a large city hospital rehabilitation center. Annually the "graduates" of the in-patient program come together to share in an afternoon of reminiscing and congratulatory support for each. These graduates, most of whom are still in outpatient care, share in their accomplishments during the previous year with the rehabilitation staff and fellow graduates. Festivities include a meal, games, prizes, and multi-media presentation of the group outings during the year.

2. I conducted personal interviews with brain-injury survivors to confirm and/or refine my findings from Preliminary Study 1, as well as to seek answers to new questions.

3. I completed a brief internship at a major trauma hospital unit to observe the initial work of the caseworker and followed acute patients in their initial impressions of injury.

Attendees at the Brain Injury Reunion were asked to complete rather lengthy questionnaires. Of the twenty-nine questionnaires completed at the reunion, twelve were completed by traumatically brain injured (TBI) patients. Participants were limited to those surviving traumatic brain injury. Individuals whose brain injury was acquired, such as stroke or tumor, were excluded from the study as they presented with some varying post brain damage characteristics, which would have made the variables to consider in analysis too great. A sample questionnaire is located in Appendix D.

Of those completing the questionnaire, four were selected for in-depth, follow-up interviews along with two other TBI patients from the trauma hospital. One of the areas of reliability weakness I noted from Preliminary Study 1 was triangulation of data. An attempt was made in Preliminary Study 2 to study medical records, speak with families, and contact therapists of those patients interviewed, where possible. The data analysis for Preliminary Study 2 followed the pattern of Preliminary Study 1.

Results

Of these 12 participants selected from those completing the questionnaire, all agreed that their struggle for a re-identification of self had been paramount. The demographic data were too widespread in this small sample to correlate any emotions with time and their struggle for re-identification post-injury. Whereas the participants in this study verified that the struggle to understand a new self was their greatest hurdle, the progression of recovery descriptions given by these survivors was enlightening. These participants seemed to agree that recovery cycled through three major stages:

1. Stage 1: Acute. The acute stage spans the time from the point of injury to the time that the individual is medically stable and ready to be discharged from his/her initial hospital stay.

2. Stage 2: Discharge. The Discharge stage begins with the discharge of the individual from his/her initial hospital stay. The entry into this stage may be as simple as discharge from the hospital to home or to a rehabilitation center, or complex like discharge home followed by an attempt to return to work. At the point of discharge, the individual is "well" and no longer considered a "patient." Now, the individual resumes life, albeit, in a new format.

3. Stage 3: Compensatory recovery. Once an individual has entered Stage 2 (Discharge) he/she discovers that his/her brain injury is for a lifetime. For some individuals, this discovery is rather sudden, for others it may be weeks, months, years until he/she realizes that some compensatory strategies must be developed to assist in routine daily activities. Once the individual realizes that he/she must compensate for his/her permanent deficits, such as short-term memory, or organizational skills he/she enters Stage 3. During this final stage of recovery, the individual develops compensatory skills to function in everyday life. For some individuals, these skills will equip him/her to reenter society and live independently; for others, the skills will allow them to function at a level sufficient for a supported community or

group home life style. Unfortunately for others, these options will never be available due to the physical extent of their injury.

These three stages as they emerged from these data are represented in Figure 3.2. Each participant recalled the length of time for passage through these stages differently; however, the progression from Stage 1 (acute) to Stage 2 (Discharge) seemed to be within the first 12 months post-injury. Progression through Stage 2 (Discharge) to Stage 3 (compensatory strategies) somewhere around the two year post-injury mark. Of the patients selected for this study, four were at least 12 months post-injury. In their retrospective analysis, each patient shared his/her feelings of "new goals" and "expectations" at the various stages as recovery progressed and their social interactions increased. An interesting phenomenon within their descriptions was that each seemed to cycle through Prochaska's five stages of change in *each* of the stages of recovery progression. That is, within each of the three recovery stages defined by the brain injured population, the patient seemed to experience the precontemplation, contemplation, preparation, action, and maintenance cycles proposed by Prochaska.

The puzzling element of their stage descriptions for me was the patients' reflection on their emotions. Generally during the acute stage (Stage 1), patients reported being at one extreme end of the emotions pendulum or the other. This extreme emotional response generally left them unable to begin the real psychological recovery, for the euphoria masked the real problems with the "it'll be all right" attitude, whereas the anger masked the real problem with the "why me" attitude. Therefore, emotions seemed to be a barrier in this first stage of progress following injury.

80

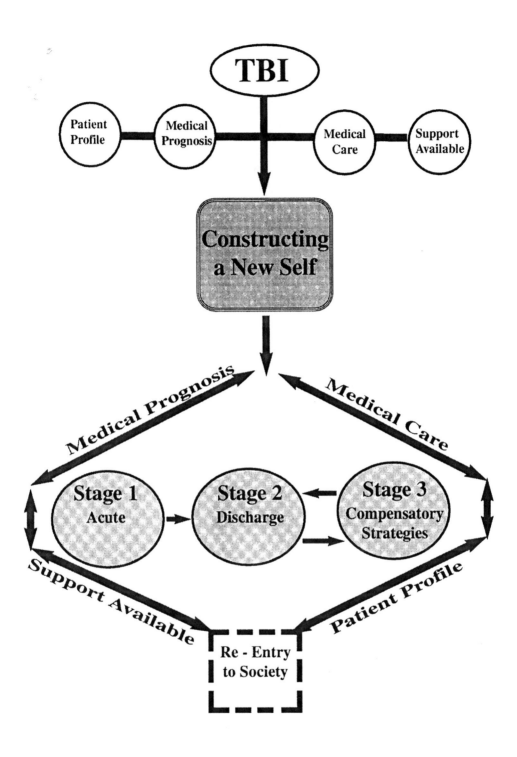

Figure 3.2.   Stages of recovery: A grounded theory model

During Stage 2, Discharge, departure from the medical setting, the patients reported that progress now could begin in earnest. During this period, patients reported they discovered the brain injury was not something that could be healed as soon as rehabilitation was over or a cast was removed, but rather that it began a period of lifelong adjustment. It was reported that during this stage, they had to reconcile the fact that compensatory strategies must be learned and then a new, albeit different, life could begin to blossom in Stage 3.

My personal observations were that this final progression stage itself had several directions: complete reentry and independent living in the community, supported community reentry, or dependent community reentry. I was intrigued with the concepts of the stages of recovery and how a patient progressed from one stage to another. Because the data was so rich in these two areas and required my full attention in order to do it justice, I abandoned the research question of technology use for this study. I did, however, question participants regarding their impressions of the usability of technology, such as e-mail support groups to get a sense of their connectedness to technology.

Discussion

Something(s) in each stage of an individual's rehabilitation progression was (were) the triggering mechanism(s) of the individuals' motivation; however, these factors remained unidentified. In all the literature reviewed, that "something" has yet to be identified, that key that turns the emotional ignition that starts the motivational engine and releases the gear for action, volition. That silent giant, I believe, is the key to understanding what motivates the TBI patient to achieve his/her greatest potential sometimes years post-injury, when the initial medical prognosis seems bleak. It was this crystallization of the ideas from patients in the two preliminary studies that led to the research questions for the dissertation, the main study. Only now, after nine months of listening to TBI patients and analyzing what they were saying, do I begin to fully appreciate the answer Sharon offered in reply to the question, "Can you define yourself now – post-injury?" "Self…for me, function and sense of self were inextricably bound together." The survivor of a traumatic brain injury seems to link his/her ability to function and his/her self-perception together.

Biased Researcher

As a participant observer, I am a biased researcher and interviewer. I have a vested interest in this topic. As explained in Chapter 1, I am TBI survivor of 13 1/2 years. It may be argued that this bias colors my research findings; I offer that my personal experience, in this case, enhances my ability to sift through the data and glean the insights about the lived experiences of being TBI survivor. During both preliminary studies, I experimented with different safety checks to prevent my overlooking rich experiences that did not match my personal experiences. I offer a review of these safety checks, my impressions, and the plan I implemented for bias protection for the main project. In Preliminary Study 1, I created and followed three rules:

1. I intentionally did not allow myself to think through my own response to any of my probes or follow-up questions. On the surface this may appear impossible, however, questions being asked such as: "Relate your progress on a timeline." or "Can you put the emotions you've experienced in an order?" require some thought. Since these are not "off the top of your head" answers as a question of "Do you ever get frustrated?" I was able to separate my own ideas and experiences and concentrate upon the participants.

2. There were many times when answers given gave me a déjà vu experience, a "matching moment." When a comment or answer caught my attention in a "matching moment" I noted it in my field book or on the audiotape. Then, when moving through the coding sequences, discussed in Chapter 4, I guarded my coding of any category until I had seen the same comment from at least three participants in the data set.

3. I was careful not to reveal to the participants before or during the interview that I, too, was a survivor. This prohibited their drawing me into conversations about shared experiences.

In Preliminary Study 1, these rules served me fairly well, except I found I missed several excellent follow-up questions because I had not thought through answers to my own questions in light of my experience. I was asking questions much as any other researcher would ask—without the inside feeling. For example, in a discussion of seizures, a patient reported that he was confused, frustrated, and sometimes angry following the episode. Those are common post-seizure emotions. A researcher without personal experience might not follow up, necessarily, with a question of "Did these feelings alter your outlook on your rehabilitation in any way?" I could have and did not in Preliminary Study 1 because I was trying so hard to avoid "contaminating" the data with my personal feelings. A better understanding of the patient's perceptions and goals, as related to the injury itself, I believe, will be a key to understanding motivational factors. Because I was interviewing on a very general level, I found no conflict of moral principle in keeping my own experience to myself. I was challenged by my qualitative research methods professor after Preliminary Study 1 with the question, "So what if they do know?" Therefore, after giving it some thought, I altered my rules for Preliminary Study 2:

1. I did think through my own questions, not in depth, but at least for recall purposes. After creating my interview questions and probes, I jotted down follow-up questions I might use if answers seemed to match my own experiences. For example, I asked the question, "How will you know when you are "recovered?" I considered my own experience and decisions I made along the way. After having been told, among other things, I would never work again, never live independently again, never be off medication, those became symbols of recovery for me. I began to define my own recovery in terms of achieving what I had been told would not happen. Therefore, when a participant offered me his/her definition of recovery, I followed up by asking what the doctor's prognosis had been originally. Then, because I have met circumstances where the doctors were right and I had to

redirect my definition of recovery, I could ask other questions. For example, I was told that I would never regain my premorbid physical stamina for activity. Promptly, I defined one area of my recovery, then, to regain personal stamina. Thirteen years post-injury, I still lack my premorbid stamina. I had to redirect my goals in order to avoid a loss of my own momentum. Therefore, based upon this experience, I was able to pursue conversations where the participants felt doomed because they were, at the time, unable to achieve one or more of their definitions of recovery.

2. I guarded against any data analysis coding of a "matching moment" on the initial entry. Like Preliminary Study 1, I waited until the third "matching moment" before labeling the category. I intentionally listened for experiences that were different to my own in order to grasp a broader understanding of the ranges of recovery possibilities.

3. I was not hesitant to share with the participants that I was TBI survivor when it came up in conversation. I did experiment in several interviews briefly sharing my survivorship as the reason for my interest in this topic prior to the interview and post interview. I was not surprised to find that in cases where I had spoken briefly of my experiences and interest in this topic prior to the interview, the answers given were more in-depth and detailed than when I remained silent on my past. While honesty in any interview relationship is important, this little experiment led me to believe that the element of self-disclosure in this interview was critical.

4. There is no escaping the fact that being a biased participant-observer is a demanding and emotionally draining experience. As a biased researcher, it would be easy to slip into total identification with the participants and miss some of the gems of information being shared if precautions are not taken to avoid such personal involvement. Therefore, I shared interview experiences with a friend who is a Ph.D., R.N. Since this friend is both a qualitative researcher and nurse she understood the importance both of my medical past emotions and the value of the data being gathered. I was able to debrief with her and separate my emotions from the data being collected.

Summary

The term "motivation" embodies many varied characteristics, any one of which offers multiple options for pursuit through research. The preliminary studies were valuable in narrowing the focus of "motivation" for the main study. Preliminary Study 1 established that the driving, or motivating, force for all survivors of traumatic brain injury is a reconstruction of self. Preliminary Study 2 confirmed the need for reconstruction of self and identified three stages of recovery: acute, discharge, and compensatory strategies. From these two preliminary studies, the area of concern for motivation in the TBI population became apparent: how does one move from stage to stage toward reconstructing self?

The guidelines established for the main study as a result of these two preliminary studies will be addressed in Chapter 4.

CHAPTER 4

METHODS FOR THE MAIN STUDY

"I like a job with a definite beginning and a definite end;
then I can see my progress"

-Stan, Windy Hill client

Introduction

While the preliminary studies illustrated varied patterns of factors influencing motivation for individuals with traumatic brain injury (TBI), there seemed to be similarities in the patterns as I watched individuals battle for recovery of function and rediscovery of self. This study sought to identify and to link these similarities through an in-depth examination of the perceptions of and methods to achieve recovery as viewed by individuals having suffered a brain injury. I elected to use a phenomenological approach and qualitative methods in which "researchers …attempt to understand the meaning of events and interactions to ordinary people in particular situations" (Bogdan & Biklen, 1992, p. 34).

In the past, research efforts studying individuals with TBI have largely been situated in the positivist paradigm, using quantitative methods, common among natural science researchers (Bergland & Thomas, 1991; Karpman, Wolfe, & Vargo, 1986; Krefting, 1990; Schacter & Crovitz, 1977). Such a paradigm has as underlying assumptions that one truth exists and that phenomena can be explained by a set of universal laws (Lincoln & Guba, 1985). Since the middle

1980's this traditional research paradigm has often been supplemented with an alternative paradigm, qualitative research. Here the researcher seeks to understand and not just explain a phenomenon, and in particular, to understand a phenomenon from within the perspectives of the individuals touched by the phenomenon. While this paradigm is not new to disciplines such as anthropology, it is relatively fresh in the field of medical research. There has been a limited number of studies of individuals with traumatic brain injury (TBI) using qualitative methods (Crisp, 1994; Hagner & Helm, 1994; Nochi, 1997; Persinger, 1993). In this chapter following the statement of problem/purpose, I will briefly discuss the characteristics of interpretivist methodology followed by the way I conducted this research study.

Statement of Problem/Purpose

I believe one of the difficulties in the study of motivational factors influencing the recovery period for rehabilitation clients is that we tend to study motivation in light of its earliest interpretations, behaviorism (Cicerone, 1989; Fugate, et.al, 1997b). While a behavior theory remains a strong foundation for the outcome indicators of the motivated client, outcome alone does not answer the perplexing question of what actually is the trigger that moves the client from idea or emotion to volition or will. I believe that an explanation of motivation lies somewhere in the relationship of our cognitive awareness to our responses to emotions. Motivation is often the term used to describe the transformation of our emotional response (feeling) to a volitional response (action). As evidenced by

90

Prigatano, this continuum is still a relatively unexplored mystery: "This appears to be in part because these two concepts have not been adequately defined and are not easily investigated in highly controlled ways. Both include an arousal component that can have reinforcing qualities." (Prigatano, in Finger, 1978, p. 348)

Therefore, this study was designed to address the following research question:

What is the genesis and nature of the motivation experienced by individuals with traumatic brain injury in rehabilitation?

The Research Approach

Following the research design of the earlier two preliminary studies, this study was conducted using qualitative methods, the details of which will be explained in four sections: the foundations of qualitative methodology, procedures employed to ensure quality of results, description of methods employed, and a discussion of the process of data collection and analysis.

Foundations of Qualitative Methodology.

I used a phenomenological approach for this study. I sought to discover the structure and the essence (Patton, 1990) of the rehabilitation experience of individuals recovering from a traumatic brain injury. Lincoln and Guba (1985) noted that in a naturalistic context, the phenomenon of interest can be studied in its own environment. A clearer understanding of motivation toward recovery for the individual with TBI must come from the environment in which rehabilitation is occurring and must occur over a period of time. Often health researchers obtain the thoughts of an individual at the point of evaluation or interview rather than over a period of time to reveal a pattern of thinking. As observed by Michael Howard, a neuropsychologist at a large rehabilitation facility, "We record the state [current action] rather than the trait [tendency]" (1998). Patterns of motivation as they relate to the progression of recovery, then, were the focus of this investigation.

One of the unique qualifiers of interpretive research traditions is the effort given to understanding the holistic nature rather than explaining a cause and effect relationship relative to a phenomenon (Strauss & Corbin, 1990). In post positivistic research, a definition of explaining a phenomenon is simply done by creating, observing, and reporting cause-effect relationships of variables. Understanding (verstehen; Lincoln & Guba, 1985) is more difficult to pinpoint. Vendler (1984) noted that when an individual allows his/her imaginations to place him/her in the other person's situation he/she may achieve understanding. Vendler challenged us not to define another's actions in objective measures, for that puts us outside the individual's intentions. Rather, Vendler concluded, to understand means to construct the story of the person's intentions as he/she connects it to his/her actions.

The goal of the phenomenological approach in qualitative research is to "understand the meaning of events and interactions to ordinary people in particular situations" (Bogdan & Biklen, 1992, p. 34). The researcher builds a structure of meanings, looking for logical rather than statistical explanations. "To the qualitative scholar, the understanding of human experience is a matter of chronologies more than of causes and effects. (Stake, 1995, p. 38). Vendler (1984) instructed those observing behavior to know the situation an individual faces if he/she is to understand the individual. The researcher cannot determine volition or intention by observing situations; but volition or intention is in relation to the situation. Each situation has as its backdrop the socio-cultural context of that time, place, participants, and event. Lincoln and Guba (1985) stated that the goal of naturalistic inquiry is verstehen, to partly understand the sociocultural context in which the person lives. Researchers do not seek to apply their preexisting ideas or thoughts to the socio-cultural context rather see it through the eyes of the participants. Describing, in depth, the processes by which individuals construct meaning are the goals of this researcher.

Evaluation Criteria and Procedural Tools to Ensure Quality.

The conventional canons of rigor associated with research are not appropriate for phenomenological inquiry. However, any intellectual inquiry must build trustworthiness if non-positivistic research is to have an impact on human knowledge (Erlandson, Harris, Skipper, & Allen, 1993). Trustworthiness can be judged in naturalistic studies such as this one by considering credibility, transferability, dependability, and confirmability (Lincoln & Guba, 1985). Each of these methodologically evaluative criteria will now be defined, and the corresponding procedures employed to ensure quality will be described, the enacting of which produces a greater likelihood of trustworthy results.

CREDIBILITY

"A central question for any inquiry relates to the degree of confidence in the 'truth' that the findings of a particular inquiry have for the subjects with which—and the context within which—the inquiry was carried out" (Lincoln & Guba, 1985, p. 290). The post-positivist paradigm establishes credibility in terms of internal validity, that is, the identical relationship between the data and the phenomena represented by those data. The non-positivist paradigm, on the other hand, examines the relationship between the realities that exist in the research participants' minds and with those ideas reconstructed by the researcher yet attributed to them (Erlandson, Harris, Skipper, & Allen, 1993). Because participants are individuals representing different realities, a credible outcome, then, is one that represents both the areas in which these realities are similar and different (Erlandson, Harris, Skipper, & Allen, 1993). I followed the series of strategies proposed by Lincoln and Guba (1985) for obtaining credibility:

• Prolonged engagement is achieved when the researcher spends enough time in the setting being studied to "overcome the distortions" (p. 301) due to his/her presence, biases, or the effects of unique events such as seasonal activities. Prolonged engagement was achieved in this study as I spent nine months working side by side with the TBI participants. Nearly 1,000 hours were spent "in the field" in the context of my participants' daily lives (Table 2). Because I was involved over such a long period of time I was able to approach an understanding of the daily events, their relationships, and the culture of the TBI rehabilitation environment. Over the span of these months I was able to observe unique events

94

such as holidays, or birthdays over several occasions thus giving insight into those areas as well.

•Persistent observation is achieved only through consistently pursuing the interpretation of events and relationships in various ways accompanied by a process of constant yet tentative analysis. For this study, persistent observation because I had the opportunity to study response to "improvement," for example, through the eyes of the TBI participant, fellow participants, often his/her family and always other staff. These various observations of the same occurrence allowed me a depth of understanding in TBIer's ability to solve or resolve a particular issue.

Table 2. Cleveland Work Log

Date	July	Aug	Sept	Oct	Nov	Dec	Jan	Feb	Mar	Apr	May
1		8	10		16	8		12			
2							15	10	8		2
3				11		8	15				
4		8		12			14				3
5		5	10		8	9	10				2**
6		5	10	8		14	6			5	1**
7		5			14	4	5	12			1**
8		4	8		14	6	7	12			2**
9					3		10	10	8		
10				11	12		12				
11				12	12		10				
12			10		12	11	12				
13			10	8	12	14	10				
14					12	12	10	10			
15		8		8	8	12	8	12			
16						10	12	8	5	6	
17				11	8	9	14			1**	
18		8				9	12			1**	
19		8	10			10				1**	
20		8	10	8				10		3	
21					10			12			
22		8			12			12			
23				6	10		12	8	5	2	
24		8	22*	8			13				
25		8		12			12	8			
26		8	10				10				
27		8	10	8						3	
28		8			8	15	8				
29		8	8		14	15					
30	3	8			12	11	12		5	1**	
31	4			16			14			1**	
Totals											1067 hours

*Overnighter
**Mini-project

•Triangulation is the term given to collecting data from different points of view. Not only are different points of view important but likewise different data sources, methods of gathering the data and different questions getting at the same answer are useful. Counter-examples are another excellent way of enhancing the strength of triangulation. Triangulation in this study was achieved by eliciting divergent constructions of the "same reality." As I gained insights into the daily routines of the clients at Epworth, I sought the supporting data, such as daily planners, posted work schedules, arrangement forms, shopping lists, PIC (personal information coordinator) reports to verify my impressions. Data that were collected from statements of participants were checked against observed behavior, participant records such as medical records, personal information coordinator reports, and daily logs. I made every attempt to arrive at alternate explanations by asking questions of different sources, and using a variety of methods to study the same event. For example, Dot once described "structure" problems concerning her work activities at and the events that occurred after she arrived back "home" (the rehabilitation group home). In order to verify the "reality," I engaged other participants in work discussion to see if I heard similar reports on "structure" concerns for workers. In addition to this, I queried the staff on the issue and their interpretation, I visited the work site, and I was "home" on occasion when Dot arrived home from work to observe for myself the problems she described. As a matter of habit upon arrival at work, I always checked the daily summary sheets for the previous 24 hours to see what events were "notable" enough to be highlighted. In addition to these triangulation efforts, I revisited participants in both preliminary studies to share the data outcome of this study and gain their opinion.

•Referential adequacy materials are data collected and set aside for examination at a later date. These data provide the opportunity to test emerging theories and models as benchmarks using analyses of data gathered earlier. The integrated interpretations of the emergent theory and the referential adequacy materials provide an adequacy check for the researcher. I frequently listened to participants as they showed me photographs from home, letters from family, gifts from family and friends. I made regular visits to their individual rooms to observe their latest "interior decorating" achievements and how they had rearranged the room or, the pride and care that they took in their personal space. Archival videotapes were made available to me for participants.

•Peer debriefing occurs when the researcher steps out of the context of his/her study and reviews perceptions, insights and analyses with professionals outside the context of the study who have enough general understanding of the context and the research to debrief the researcher. The purpose of peer debriefing is for the researcher to refine and/or redirect the inquiry process. Peer debriefing was implemented often during the course of this project. I contracted with Barbara Holmes, Ph.D., R.N., a peer health care worker, to debrief at three specific points in data analysis. The first debriefing took place in mid-January with a visit to the sites and lengthy discussion of my observations. Barbara observed my interactions with the participants and discussions took place on the benefits of actions as well as areas that could be improved upon. The second debriefing with Barbara came in mid-February when all categories had been named and relationships were being formulated amongst them. References in the transcriptions were checked and discussed for validity of interpretation and suggestions were made for additional category refinement. The final debriefing by Barbara occurred in late March after the final model had been completed.

In addition to this health care colleague, Esther, my transcriptionist, and I engaged in bi-monthly discussions of possible interpretations and relationships. Prior to finalizing my grounded theory, I spent several sessions with various traumatic brain injury rehabilitation staff sharing ideas, and my view of emerging relationships in the data.

Due to the intensity of the potential personal emotional impact of this research, I debriefed weekly with my dissertation supervisor. Other members of my committee were contacted as their area of expertise was needed in analysis. A preliminary draft of the dissertation was sent to the members of the committee as a check for any contextual "holes" that needed to be repaired prior to leaving the research site. In addition to the interval checking completed with members of my committee, the manuscript and findings were checked and critiqued by three professors of research, and three members of the brain injury rehabilitation profession.

•Member checks allow the participants to have a voice in the interpretation of the data. Seeking the verification of my interpretations of events with my TBI population was perhaps the most exciting of all credibility "quality check" tools for me. Due to the nature of this research and the rapport I was fortunate to develop with my participants I would often "check" my theories and ideas with them. An interesting phenomenon actually grew from member checks. After six months I had several "group interviews" to seek additional information. Following the conclusion of these group interviews, in future weeks as I would be "member checking" with one participant, before I knew it there were usually five or six more discussants. It was interesting to watch their pride that the interpretations were accurate and that they did, in fact, have a voice. In the latter weeks of my involvement, participants requested we continue our "research meetings."

In addition to the member checking of the participants in this study, participants from both preliminary studies were consulted and given opportunity to validate the findings. It was apparent that these earlier participants were pleased to see the foundation contributions that they had made. Without exception, the findings were validated by earlier participants, both in personal interview and revisiting on-line participants.

TRANSFERABILITY

"An inquiry is judged in terms of the extent to which its findings can be applied in other contexts or with other respondents" (Lincoln & Guba, 1985, p. 290). In traditional study it is the researcher's responsibility to ensure that findings can be generalized to the population; in a naturalistic study the responsibility for demonstrating transferability rests with those who would apply the findings to another context (Lincoln & Guba, 1985). Transferability is enhanced by the researcher in two ways:

•Thick description brings the reader vicariously into the context being described. Because transferability is dependent upon the similarities of sending and receiving the contexts, the researcher strives to collect detailed descriptions of data in context and report them with sufficient detail and precision to allow the reader a vicarious experience. Thick description even includes specific details such as sights, sounds, relationships in the context being studied. Thick description was my goal as I wrote not only my field notes but also the goal of my transcriptionist as she interpreted the sounds and "atmosphere" she heard on tape. On the audiotape I often would give her a detailed description of the incident in analysis which she transcribed for depth of understanding. It was my goal in writing this dissertation to provide a vicarious experience for the reader.

•Purposive sampling seeks to maximize the range of specific information about the context. I made efforts to have systematic and widespread theoretical sampling (Strauss & Corbin, 1990) by means of the varied demographic nature of the participant population. For example, there was a wide age range, there were multiple injury diagnoses and personal prognoses, and premorbid characteristics represented a cross-section of the general population.

DEPENDABILITY

In naturalistic inquiry the researcher must provide his/her audience with evidence that if the study were repeated with the same or similar participants (subjects) in the same (or a similar) context, the findings would be similar if not repeated (Lincoln & Guba, 1985).

> In the traditional research paradigm this dependability is spoken of in terms of reliability, which of course speaks of the predictability, stability, or accuracy of the research 'instrument.' In the traditional paradigm one cannot achieve validity without reliability, that is, an assumption of

isomorphic relationships between observation and reality cannot be made if replication yields different results. To the qualitative researcher, on the other hand, any differences in relationships may not only be 'error' but more importantly shifts in reality. Therefore, the quest for the qualitative researcher is not 'invariance' but for 'trackable variance' (Guba, 1981 as cited in Erlandson, Harris, Skipper, & Allen, 1993, p. 34).

Therefore, qualitative "reliability" is conceived in terms of "dependability," that is, can changes in the data and interpretation be "tracked." Guba suggested that a dependability audit embraces both the stability implied by "reliability" and the trackability required by explainable changes (1981, p. 81). A dependability audit trail was created for this study through careful documentation of dates, times, places of incidents and cross-referenced through interview notes, field notes, and site documents such as daily logs, etc.

CONFIRMABILITY

Finally, according to Lincoln and Guba, "an inquiry is judged in terms of the degree to which its findings are the product of the focus of its inquiry and not of the biases of the researcher" (1985, p. 290). For the traditional researcher, attempts are made to insulate observations from the biases of the researcher and provide replicable results. The qualitative researcher acknowledges that "objectivity is an illusion and actually no methodology can be totally separated from those who have created and selected it"(Erlandson, Harris, Skipper, & Allen, 1993, p. 34). Therefore, I sought not to ensure that my observations were free from "personal bias contamination" but rather to offer data that could be tracked to their sources, and interpretations that were logical and structurally coherent.

Following the guidelines established by Guba and Lincoln (1989, p. 243) I established a confirmability audit trail. Prior to finalizing my grounded theory model, I sought the outside audit of my data sources and interpretation by two of my committee members, my health care colleague, my transcriptionist, and two seasoned veterans of the rehabilitation network. I selected these six for this audit since I felt they represented the academic, medical, general public, and brain injury rehabilitation audiences respectively.

Trustworthiness, though important, is not sufficient alone as a measure of the quality of the results of the study. The quality of the results is measured also by the benefits gained by the participants. This is called authenticity. There are five authenticity criteria: fairness, and the authenticity of ontological, educative, catalytic, and tactical natures. Each will be reviewed briefly and illustrated in light of this study.

•Fairness - Informed consent should be obtained from participants at the very beginning of the research project and should be renewed continuously throughout the project. This periodic renewal throughout the research protects the power relationship of participant/researcher since in human contexts relationships and/or desires may continually shift. This criterion allows the participant the freedom to withdraw at any time during the research. This flexibility, of course, is anathema to the traditional researcher who believes such matters are handled prior to the study once and for all. In this study, prior to any contact with participants, the design was approved by the Epworth Rehabilitation Network Board of Education, and the University of Texas Institutional Review Board. Following this approval, participant consent was obtained. Throughout the daily contact individuals were often reminded that they had the freedom not to answer, or to withdraw entirely from the project.

•Ontological authenticity enables the participants to understand their world better with reference to the focus of the study, in this case, recovery. Participants gain the ability, as a result of their participation, to see the larger picture of their world. Individuals often gain the ability to be reflective upon their interactions as a result of ontological soundness. This was illustrated in my study when Richard gained valuable insight into the procedures needed for planning a move to the apartments. Richard had been anxious to progress in his recovery, however, in setting his goals for making the move to the apartments, he failed to set the preliminary goals at each achievement level such as, budgeting to have extra money at the end of each month to put in savings for his first month rent. As a result of our discussions and his interactions with other clients in this project, Richard began to realize the nature of his own planning stages in any project.

•Educative authenticity for me is one of the most important criterion for it speaks to the importance of "each one, teach one." Educative authenticity is achieved when the participants are able to effectively share their new knowledge gained with others. In my study, this happened a multitude of times. One of the greatest compliments I received came from Ellis who shared with me,

> You know, after all these months of listening to how you think as a TBIer, I've learned to do it myself. But the neatest thing was when Grace was in trouble the other day and I told her some of the things we talked about and she tried it and solved the problem. So, I decided that I have the advantage helping these new guys since I'm a TBIer and can help them. I like that. So all those mornings we cooked breakfast together, paid off.

•Catalytic authenticity occurs when the participants become inspired to participate and be involved in activities in their lives related to new knowledge gained by participating in the study. I was fortunate to have no problem seeing this authenticity played before my very eyes. There is a very fine line between catalytic authenticity and tactical authenticity as illustrated below.

•Tactical authenticity is illustrated by the extent to which the participants act upon what they have learned. The ongoing project with Darrell that evolved from this research is illustrative of this criterion. From the principles Darrell gained as a participant in this research exhibiting catalytic authenticity, he has gained planning skills and the initiative to be more involved in his nursery work. He is now building a stronger future in his nursery work because he is now planning and organizing his work at the nursery, evidence of tactical authenticity. Therefore, catalytic authenticity is the inspiration; tactical authenticity is the perspiration.

Description of Study

As no *a priori* theory exists for the progression of recovery from TBI or the motivational factors involved, the Strauss and Corbin (1990) method of generating models with grounded theory was best suited to this study. Limited descriptive quantitative data were used as supporting evidence for conclusions drawn. In addition, due to the large amount of data gathered from two sites, some quantitative coding was required simply to organize the data. This study was carried out at two sites with confirming data gathered from both an on-line TBI electronic mail discussion list, and from participants involved in both earlier studies. The processes I used for this project will be presented in five sections: (1) site description; (2) participant selection criteria; (3) data source identification; (4) participant observer activities at each site; and (5) data analysis process.

Site Description

The search for a data gathering site began with a visit to the World Wide Web home page of the national Brain Injury Association of America (BIAA), URL: http://www.biausa.org/, as well as phone calls to various traumatic brain injury rehabilitation specialists across the country. I also sought the counsel of state BIAA directors regarding the rehabilitation facilities available that might welcome a research project. Following leads and advice from these sources, I created a list of over a dozen places to visit. Recognized rehabilitation specialists had provided introductions for me, so I had no difficulty in obtaining appointments to explore the research opportunities. After spending two months touring various facilities while conducting my second preliminary study, I selected a large rehabilitation center, Epworth, in a small university town of 150,000 residents. The university had some contact with the rehabilitation network, therefore, research was welcome.

ABOUT THE EPWORTH REHABILITATION NETWORK

Epworth Rehabilitation Network offered a comprehensive continuum of care through nine interrelated treatment facilities. The network facilities are located within a 25-mile radius of the small university community. Epworth's program offered each individual with a traumatic brain injury (hereafter called client) a supportive transition from a highly structured behavioral rehabilitation program to a moderately structured vocational program to a less structured, community-based, reentry program. These gradations in rehabilitation available allowed each client to progress at his/her own pace. All nine treatment facilities within the Epworth network followed the same philosophy of treatment. Therefore, prior to a discussion of my specific site-related activities, I will offer an overview of the Epworth network focusing upon the major common factors of daily structure, the color-category-driven token economy, and Rutledge Review Days.

The Epworth treatment programs are grounded in the belief that all individuals feel good about themselves when they are productive. Activities were structured at each of the facilities from 6:30 a.m. – 9:30 p.m. The daily activities of clients included participation in personalized therapeutic programs, academic programs, and vocational programs. The evening activities offered structured leisure, individual or group outings in the community such as bowling, sporting events, movies, dining out, theatre, or seasonal activities. Each activity was designed with a therapeutic purpose in mind. Staff members were responsible for one to three clients at a time, depending upon the supervision needs of the clients. Each staff member was encouraged to be a role model and work alongside the client rather than watching him/her work, with the goal of generating a supportive growth environment rather than the traditional clinical staff-patient relationship. As discovered in Preliminary Study 1, the struggle to redefine self following brain injury is paramount in recovery and fraught with emotional unrest. The rehabilitation approach of Epworth allowed individuals to begin feeling successful from their first day with the program as they rediscovered life.

Epworth uses a token economy system to allow the clients to achieve monetary rewards for each accomplishment, such as completing their exercise program, participating in academic activities, completing housekeeping chores, or demonstrating appropriate behavior. Following a brain injury, individuals often feel they are of "no value" because they are not "doing regular things" or "earning a living" (Nochi, 1997). The token economy system offered each client the opportunity to be successful daily. A client would then use his/her earnings to pay for personal items and outings. Clients were encouraged to earn enough to pay for room and board by the month as they progressed through the system. Although the actual payment for room and board was covered in the per diem fee for each client, the feeling of earning one's way by paying token money for room and board was designed to increase the growth of self-esteem. The recovery process following traumatic brain injury is different for each individual, but the need for feeling good about one's self is the same for all (Nochi, 1997).

As a client progressed in his/her recovery, he/she was offered the ability to work and earn a living. Epworth owned and operated five different businesses that provided on site vocational training for the clients. Each program allowed for increasing challenges that clients could begin at a basic level of work responsibility and earn their way up to more complex responsibilities. Epworth also offered a community reentry program in which clients learned independent living skills for day-to-day life. Unlike the primary programs where clients lived in a dorm-like setting, clients progressing to the level of the community reentry program lived initially in a small supervised group home, then advanced to their own apartment, usually shared with one other client. At the community reentry level of participation, the clients could take advantage of the educational opportunities of the community, such as the local high school and university. For the clients who were not able to achieve independent living, Epworth offered a long-term residential rehabilitation program. The focus of these programs was to develop treatment plans that concentrated upon a quality and productive lifestyle in the least restrictive environment possible. It was the philosophy of Epworth that each client could continue to progress in a supportive environment.

Privileges within the token economy system were gained as the clients advanced through a sequence of colors. Based upon the rainbow, the color categories were the cornerstone for progress through the system of the rehabilitation network. The purpose of the color categories was to teach the budgeting process as well as to boost self-esteem through achievement. As the client moved through the color system, he/she was able to move from token to real dollars. Each color category had characteristics common to that color, such as "the client is proficient at carrying and logging information in a daily diary," or "clients have achieved success in paying for their room by the week." As a client moved up in the rainbow of colors, more privileges were offered, such as number of phone calls that could be made, or outings that could be earned, or television time that could be available. A client was not eligible for consideration for a move to the community reentry program until he/she had earned at least the distinction of the "blue" category, four steps removed from the entry level color.

"Payday" (held at the conclusion of each day) in the Epworth token economy was based upon 1/3 participation, 1/3 attitude, and 1/3 achievement of targeted treatment objectives. The staff's assessment of the client's success in each of those three areas determined the percentage of his/her hourly wage earned each hour during the day. For example, a client could have a terrific morning and receive "full pay" (based on his/her color category, beginning at $4.00/hour), yet then have a behavioral outburst and receive no pay for a couple of hours in the afternoon. He/she could earn his/her way "back into the structure" and regain near to or full pay in the evening hours.

Prior to admission, each client was evaluated by the Epworth staff and consultations were made with all concerned parties in the client's rehabilitation history. Individualized programs were developed for each client within the overall structure of the system. These rehabilitation plans were designed, with the client, by the team of occupational therapists, physical therapists, physicians, teachers, and program managers along with family members and medical team members. Upon admission, each client's program was tailor-made for his/her needs. While the day-to-day operation was conducted at each of the nine facilities by separate staff members, the continuity of the Epworth philosophy and monitoring of each client's progress was checked every three weeks. This was a process conducted by the corporate management team, consisting of the Chief Executive Officer and Medical Director, Dr. Rutledge; the neuropsychologist, Dr. Bates; the clinical director, Mr. Starnes; and the case manager, Ms. Ketchum (all pseudonyms). These days of review for each client were called "Rutledge Review Days." On these days, the corporate management team traveled to each site and spent the day on location. The events of that day would include a preview meeting at 7:30 a.m. involving the review team and the facility's leadership. Leadership team members would offer a brief review and update of each client's accomplishments during the past three week, medical concerns, goals, and problem areas. Following this meeting, each client would have an individual meeting of 30-45 minutes chaired by one of the four members from the corporate team. Also attending the client's meeting would be his/her facility staff PIC (personal information co-ordinator) as well as any family or personal case managers interested. With this group, the clients had the opportunity to receive feedback, express likes, dislikes, questions, or just chat. Clients were paid (token money) by the corporate staff for each goal they achieved during the three-week period. The corporate member utilized this time to reinforce the direction of the treatment program and assess any areas of change that were merited. Following the morning of individual meetings, they enjoyed lunch with staff, clients, and families interacting and socializing. Clients returned to their regular afternoon schedules while facility staff and the corporate management team gathered to debrief on each client and discuss any program changes needed. These review days offered a consistent, comprehensive, and regular update of each client's progress and aided in the discharge planning that would begin weeks prior to discharge.

Selection Criteria for Participants

Four categories of participants contributed to this study: individuals with a traumatic brain injury, rehabilitation staff members, families of individuals with a traumatic brain injury, and myself, the investigator, as participant observer.

INDIVIDUALS WITH TRAUMATIC BRAIN INJURY

A total of 64 individuals who had suffered a traumatic brain injury were observed over a period of nine months for this study. After Preliminary Study 2, I decided to limit this study to individuals with traumatic brain injury, thereby excluding any individuals with a congenital or degenerative brain injury. While many of the rehabilitation techniques are similar for both populations, the emotional impact of the trauma appeared to me to generate different motivational traits; therefore, an effort was made to control as far as possible the initiating factors that might contribute to the motivation of the individual. Traumatic brain injury was selected in preference to congenital or degenerative brain injury because I had first-hand knowledge of it, and because it is an area with increasing interest in the field of neurological rehabilitation. I spent portions of one week discussing my research ideas and goals with various management team members from Epworth. Participants were then identified by the Chief Executive Officer, the Clinical Director, the Staff Neuropsychologist, and the Education Committee of Epworth Rehabilitation Network. The selection was carried out in this manner because Epworth holds the legal rights for protection of confidentiality for each resident. This method of participant identification was in compliance with the guidelines presented by the Institutional Review Board of The University of Texas at Austin. With the exception of six, the participants were all residents of either the Windy Hill or the Tallangatta programs (Tables 3 & 4). The remaining six were all clients whom I worked with at one of the network vocational sites.

<u>Table 3</u>. Windy Hill Clients

TBI Client	Sex	Age at Intv	Injury Age	Years Before Admis	Other Rehab	Cause	Edu. Level	Time w P-O
Richard	M	32	21	4		MVA	HS+2	3
Todd	M	26	15	8	YES	MV-B	hs	5
Peggy	F	27	23	3		MVA	hs	5
Myrtle	F				NO	MVA	HS	5
Stan	M	34	19	14	YES	MVA	HS+2	5
Grant	M	51	40	1		Work	HS	3
Kyle	M	35	18	5	NO	MVA	HS	3
Chip	M	22	5	12	YES	Home	GED+	3
Jeff	M	49	29	2		Work	hs	4
Fred	M	21	20	-	NO	Home	hs	5
Milton	M	43	27	-	NO	MVA	GED	4
Joe	M	31	15	8	YES	MV-P	hs	3
Wally	M	22	21	1	NO	MVA	HS	5
Mack	M	30	17	4		MVA	hs	3
Don	M	31	18	9		MVA	hs	3
Len	M	20	18	1	NO	MVA	GED	5
EC	M	52	35	5			hs	5
Ruth	F	52	33	3		MVA	HS+2	4
Jerome	M	43	31	9	YES	MV-P	HS	3
Benjie	M	32	26	1		MV-P	GED	3
Hunter	M	28	16	7		Home	Hs	4
Ryan	M	42	30	2	YES	MVA	GED+	
Greg	M	58	42	2		MVA	HS	3
Dave	M	26	25	-	NO	MVA	HS	5
Joey	M	21	19	-	NO	MVA	HS	1
Troy	M	24	23	-	NO	Work	HS+2	1
Thomas	M	26	24	2	YES	MVA	HS	2

Legend:
Cause: MVA = Motor Vehicle Accident; MV-P = Car/pedestrian;
              MV-B = Car/Bike; Home = accident in or around home; Work = hurt
              on job
Education: HS = high school graduation; hs = less than high school education;
              GED = diploma; GED+ = college hours beyond GED; GED+2 = 2
              years beyond GED
P=O (participant-observer) time: 1 = minimal; 2 = short; 3 = average (most
staff time); 4 = more than average; 5 = extensive

Table 4. Tallangatta Clients

TBI Client	Sex	Age at Intv	Injury Age	Years Before Admis	Other Rehab	Cause	Edu. Level	Time w P-O
Rod	M	18	12	3	YES	MV-P	hs	3
Ray	M	44	26	10	YES	MVA	HS+5	5
Grace	F	36	21	9	YES	MVA	HS	3
Joy	F	27	15	4	YES	MV-P	GED	5
Cecilia	F	23	12	9	YES	Home	HS	5
Allan	M	20	18	1	YES	MVA	HS	4
Paula	F	25	18	1	YES	MVA	HS	4
Loren	M	28	26	2	YES	MVA	HS	3
Wally	M	22	21	1/2	NO	MVA	HS	5
Tim	M	45	38	1/2	NO	Work	HS	5
Neal	M	31	20	6	YES	MVA	HS	3
Terri	F	30	27	1	YES	MVA	HS	5
Darrell	M	34	22	5	YES	MV-P	HS	5
Ellis	M	38	24	3	YES	MVA	HS	5
Hugh	M	36	20	3	YES	MVA	HS+2	5
Ernest	M	39	28	-	NO	MVA	HS	4
Ronnie	M	40	32	4	NO	Work	HS	4
Clyde	M	19	9	7	YES	MVA	hs	4
Freddie	M	25	16	2	YES	MVA	HS	3
Don	M	41	31	1	NO	MVA	HS	4
Thomas	M	31	15	8	YES	MVA	HS+1	3
Harold	M	19	12	3	NO	MVA	hs	4
Jim	M	33	19	2	YES	MV-P	HS	4
Stu	M	35	21	4	YES	Work	HS	3
Ruben	M	56	46	1/2	NO	Work	HS	3
Mildred	F	56	44	2 1/2	YES	Work	HS	5
Ruben	M	47	15	20	YES	Home	HS	5

Legend:
Cause: MVA = Motor Vehicle Accident; MV-P = Car/pedestrian;
            MV-B = Car/Bike; Home = accident in or around home; Work = hurt
            on job
Education: HS = high school graduation; hs = less than high school education;
            GED = diploma; GED+ = college hours beyond GED; GED+2 = 2
            years beyond GED
P=O time: 1 = minimal; 2 = short; 3 = average (most staff time); 4 = more than
            average; 5 = extensive

Eligibility criteria for the participants were as follows: older than 16 years of age, a pathologically confirmed diagnosis of traumatic brain injury, no history of drug or alcohol abuse or psychiatric illness, medically stable with a GOAT (Galveston Orientation and Awareness Test) score of at least 75, and fluency in English. In the early stages of the study it had been my intent to exclude participants who had suffered an open head injury; however, after observing potential participants carefully for months, I elected to include open as well as closed head injuries because once medically stable, they seemed to respond in a similar manner to each other.

Approval was obtained from the Departmental Review Committee of the Department of Educational Psychology, The University of Texas at Austin; The University of Texas at Austin Institutional Review Board and the Education Committee and the Board of Directors of the Epworth Rehabilitation Network. I was most fortunate to have the undivided attention of the Epworth corporate management team in the early days of this project. Their attention to detail as well as to my research goals provided the foundation for positive experiences at each of the facilities with which I would come in contact during the next nine months. I was given full support and encouragement for this investigation.

After the research plans had been reviewed and approved and I had received basic training in orientation sessions, I reported for duty at the Rotation 1 site, Windy Hill. My responsibilities and activities will be discussed in detail later in this chapter.

While my researcher status was not made a focal point in my introduction to the clients at each site, all participants were made aware of my investigator status and contributed on a voluntary basis. Each participant received careful explanation of my research focus and was frequently reminded of their freedom of choice to withdraw from any discussion at any time. For clients' protection, all names used in this dissertation are pseudonyms.

Rehabilitation Staff Members

While I observed more than five dozen staff members, exclusive of corporate team members, I worked closely with 35 and of those, became "close" to 14. Staff members ranged in age from 21 – 62 and in educational level from GED (General Education Diploma) to Master's degrees. Several staff members were enjoying this position as a retirement avocation, meaning they had retired from another job in education, the military or business. Many staff members were graduates of the local university with a Bachelor's degree, having completed the internship for their degree working at the Epworth network. Again, my status as participant observer was made clear to the staff and they were assured of their freedom to withhold any opinion or research participation. Staff were periodically reassured of the confidentiality of their opinions with regard to my sharing specific information with the administration of the Epworth network that might endanger their jobs. For staffers' protection, all names used in this dissertation are pseudonyms and at times, even the gender and age have been changed for privacy.

Families of Individuals with a Traumatic Brain Injury

Often family members or friends of the Epworth residents would attend periodic system-wide review sessions or visit the facilities. As the opportunity presented itself, I would interview family members. These interviews were really more directed conversations than interviews, because I wanted to gain an understanding of their opinions without concerning them that their loved one was being "watched" or "studied." On four occasions when I met family members, they were most responsive because their family member had told them of our friendship and work together. With these families, I had the opportunity to visit on a number of occasions during the period of this study. There were an additional five families and friends with whom I had opportunity for contact. For families' protection, all names used in this dissertation are pseudonyms.

Investigator as Participant Observer

As noted in Chapters 1 and 3, I am a biased researcher by virtue of my own traumatic brain injury in 1984. Having reviewed the steps I tried in each of the Preliminary Studies to be conscious of researcher bias, these are the safeguards I decided upon in this study:

1. I thought through my own questions and probes according to my experience; and used them to guide me in forming in-depth probes for more detailed answers.

2. I made a conscious attempt to discover experiences that did not match any of my own to ensure that I had explored a wide variety of experiences.

3. I sought to be on guard for isolated "matching moments" (déjà vu experiences) by listening for said moment at least three times.

4. As I discovered, especially in Preliminary Study 2, reliving some of my own TBI experiences was emotionally and physically draining, I regularly sought to debrief my own feelings and frustrations with my Ph.D., R.N. friend as well as my dissertation supervisor. I made a conscious effort to withdraw for short periods of time to safeguard against my personal recollection clouding my analysis.

5. I was honest and open with participants and I believe it enhanced the quality and depth of their answers. I did not, however, offer my own experiences in such a manner as to be drawn into a comparison discussion.

While these five guidelines did serve me well, I had no way of knowing how emotionally draining this study would be. Unlike the Preliminary Studies, I was immersed for hours at a time in the actual rehabilitation setting. Often in the early days and weeks, I was torn between the "me" that was the staff member, the "me" that was the researcher, and the "me" that had been just where my participants were. At times I experienced flashbacks of my own rehabilitation emotions such as hurt, anger, frustration, confusion, or anxiety. While I did withdraw from situations that were hurtful and painful reminders at times, the experience was still emotive. I cannot count the nights I drove home from work/data-gathering fighting back tears as I thought about the day's activities and relived my own experiences. After approximately 5 1/2 weeks in Rotation 1, I felt secure and only occasionally had the isolated flashback moment. Happily approaching Rotation 2, I was unaware of the coming revival of these flashbacks. I falsely assumed that I had "conquered" these feelings during Rotation 1. However, because the change in Rotation represented a change in the level of functioning of the participants, I entered the emotional flashbacks of my own rehabilitation anew and at another level. Fortunately, like Rotation 1, after a few weeks, I was able to distance myself and only experienced the occasional flashback.

While one certainly does not have to experience a traumatic brain injury to be an effective rehabilitation support member, I do believe that the flip side of the weakness of my being a biased researcher holds one of the major strengths of this study. Motivation is a difficult concept to grasp at best, let alone its expression confounded by the struggle of the individual with a brain injury. However, having experienced some of the same struggles and emotions as my informants, I could better identify the motivational factors and ramifications for my participants as they occurred. Furthermore, there is absolutely no doubt that my having experienced a brain injury gave me "instant credibility" with my participants when they learned of my injury. This led to an unspoken camaraderie privileged and understood only among TBI survivors.

Summary of Data Sources

In interpretative inquiry, it is important to give attention to the construction of a comprehensive, holistic portrayal of the socio-cultural dimensions of the research setting. Each individual, site, event, artifact is considered a unique entity with its own particular meanings and constellation of relationships emerging from the socio-cultural context in which it was found (Patton, 1990). There are four general sources of data used by the researcher of natural inquiry: interviews, observation, documents, and artifacts (Erlandson, Harris, Skipper, & Allen, 1993). Data was obtained from each of these sources for this study.

INTERVIEWS

1.　Audiotaped daily activities and interviews

During Rotation 1, I audiotaped daily activities, including all conversation, throughout the day and on multiple occasions. I wore a lavaliere microphone with a Sony TCM-59V voice-activated cassette recorder attached to my belt. In addition to recording the daily activities, I conducted ten semi-structured interviews. For these interviews, I met with the participants in four groupings (3,3,2,2). I chose this small grouping arrangement for interviews for three reasons:

(1)　I could arrange to be assigned to particular clients during noon time and conduct the interviews during this time; therefore, not interrupting their structure,

121

(2)   the time required of me for individual interviews would have burdened others as my responsibilities as a staff member would have gone unattended during those hours, and

(3)   in a group setting the clients were less apprehensive.

During the group interviews, I would ask a question, all participants would respond, then the group would engage in a discussion of the topic. Following my planned questions, I provided time for the participants to discuss any motivational matter of concern or interest to them.

In the initial minutes of each group interview, the facility manager met with us and spoke to the clients of his approval and support for their honest opinion, reassuring them that neither he nor any Epworth employee would be hearing any of the tapes. He explained that following the completion of this study, all tapes would be destroyed. He assured the participants that they had no reason for concern of retaliation in any form and encouraged them to participate actively, as their opinions could be of help to others having suffered a traumatic brain injury. This verbal support established a very positive tone for honest, in-depth discussions. Following his announcement, the manager left the room in order to give the participants complete freedom to express themselves.

Audiotaping during Rotation 2 was limited to individual or small group interviews, as the participants at this level were not comfortable during the day with their comments being recorded. Their reasons for concern actually evolved from the knowledge that I, too, was a TBI survivor, and often the participants desired to engage in personal conversations of their concerns, seeking my opinion. In my role as the staff member assisting them, I felt it important to allow all these conversations to be private. In cases in which a topic was mentioned that I thought might have bearing on the motivational factors, I made a note in my field book and revisited the issue when we were "on record" and the participant was aware that he/she was being recorded. Primarily due to the nature of the daily structure (schedule) at the Tallangatta program, I did not have the luxury of staff encouragement prior to interviews. Fortunately, the cognitive/physical level of functioning of the participants in this program did not require staff support to share their opinions. In addition to daily activities and interviews, several Rutledge Review Days were taped during both rotations, and some personal field notes were taped in addition to my written field notes. Examples of the taped field notes are observations during Rutledge Review Days, activities on group outings, events occurring at the woodshop or nursery.

2.   Client Interviews

In addition to the formal interviews that were audiorecorded, I made copious notes on participant discussions in my field books. I usually noted environmental observations as well as personal observations about the participant when entering discussion information.

3.   Staff Interviews

Informally, I interviewed, and likewise discussed motivational factors with the 14 staff I knew well. These interviews were not recorded other than in my field notebook. I chose only to enter these conversations in my field book because I discovered that when I focused our conversations upon my internship and my interest in learning as opposed to questioning as a researcher, I gained much more information and staff insights. While the staff were always willing to share, they appeared to be less threatened and more communicative teaching a participant intern than an observant researcher. My data from the rehabilitation workers were centered around the task at hand. I attempted "thick description" each time I entered some observation of health care worker behavior that I felt affected motivational factors of the client.

4.   Family Interviews

As previously discussed, I enjoyed communicating with the family and friends of the participants when given the opportunity to do so. None of these interviews were recorded other than in my field book, because family opinions were supportive data and not the focus of this study and I sought not to cause any reason for concern among visiting family members by asking too many questions.

OBSERVATION

5. Rutledge Review Days

I attended all Rutledge Review Days while I worked in each Rotation. On many occasions, I attended the Rutledge Day for the opposite facility in order to keep abreast of the progress of my clients and any motivational factors that had arisen. The method of recording these data were varied: actual meeting recordings that were transcribed, field notes, copies of Rutledge Day documentation (PIC reports), follow-up conversations with individual clients. The method for collecting these data was dependent upon the tone of the day when I arrived at the site.

6.   Field notes

My activities over the nine months were recorded in 4 8 1/2" x 11" hardbound notebooks. Personal handwritten notes produced data totaling just over 400 pages.

DOCUMENTS

7.   Transcriptions

A total of 64 hours of data were recorded and transcribed. These recordings yielded approximately 550 pages of transcription. Dialogue was single-spaced with blank lines inserted between speakers. I was fortunate to have a transcriptionist, Esther, who was not only fast, but accurate in recording detail. Esther maintained a tight turn-around time on tapes that allowed me the luxury of quick transcription review for follow-up inquiries or attention to certain details. In addition to her accuracy, Esther entered valuable information such as lengthy pauses, asides, environmental distractions that may have been present, or tone of voice if there were sudden changes. Though I listened to each tape at least three times prior to its transcription, these additional comments were helpful in data analysis. Esther also offered insights of participant growth from her own view listening to the tapes; events I had not necessarily connected. For example, one day, during morning Physical Exercises, I asked Peggy to assist me by going to get a change of blouses for Martha. Upon returning, Peggy explained her selection due to the cold temperature. She said, "Since it's cold outside, I brought a long-sleeved shirt." Esther noted that to her, this was a great example of Peggy's growth intellectually over the months: she actually had thought about the best choice of tops for Martha.

8.   Videotapes

Epworth maintained a videotape history of most of their clients. This archival information was made available to me. As the research project neared its conclusion, I revisited the tapes for the primary participants and made pertinent data entries in my field books. For example, periodically a client may be videotaped by one of the Epworth videographers during an arrangement meeting to capture his/her interpersonal communication skills. By viewing tapes that had been edited with months, often years, in between, progress of reaching goals and change in behavior was visible.

9.   Medical Records

Complete medical records of each participant were made available to me. I recorded pertinent data such as nature of injury, date of injury, age at injury and, date of Epworth admission.

ARTIFACTS

10.   Archival Information

All documentation on client progress was recorded at the Central Office for the Epworth network. I was given opportunity and assistance to peruse the files of personal information coordinator sheets, accident reports, progress reports, and more for each client. In addition to the client data, all rehabilitation data such as color categories, token economy earnings, and staff procedures/policies were made available. Archival documentation selected totaled over 200 pages of additional data.

11. FTP Questionnaire

One of the advantages of grounded theory strategies is that the constant comparative method of data analysis allows the researcher to make comparisons, then ask follow-up questions for additional information, then compare again. The experiences gained in the preliminary studies allowed me to be prepared to take advantage of this unique process. Beginning in the first week I analyzed data through comparison and questioning. For example, approximately six weeks into data gathering I noticed that a client appeared to work harder on his/her rehabilitation programs when conversations had just been held discussing his/her future. That is, how a client perceived his/her future seemed to influence his/her rehabilitation work energies. After observing this property of the motivational phenomenon, I shared the idea with a graduate colleague, Jenefer Husman, whose dissertation research focused on a concept labeled, Future Time Perspective (FTP) (1998). Basically, the concept as defined by L.K. Frank stated "actions, emotions, and certainly the morale of an individual at any instant depends upon his total time perspective" (Lewin, 1942, p. 48-49). Husman's research led to the development of an instrument to measure the FTP as it relates to the motivation of an average college-aged population. Husman and I collaborated altering her trial instrument for my traumatically brain injured population. The questionnaire, administered twice, at two month intervals, to individuals in both facilities where I worked is found in Appendix A.

Participant Observer Activities at Each Site

ROTATION 1

My first field experience rotation took place in one of the mid-level facilities, Windy Hill. The clientele at this facility fluctuated between 18 – 24 residents, mostly men. The ratio of men to women followed the national ratio of 4 – 1 men to women with head injury. The age span of residents at this facility was 18 – 52 years. Six clients were lifelong residents while the remainder were transitional. Most often, clients had been oriented to the Epworth rehabilitation structure at another facility prior to transfer to Windy Hill. Clients progressing to the Windy Hill program usually did not have major behavioral problems (although they may still have had some occasional and/or minor problems) and were ready to begin some type of vocational training. Vocational work for the clients in this program was always within the Epworth network-owned and-operated businesses.

The corporate management team requested that, in return for gathering data at their facilities, I undergo all preemployment testing and training of a regular staff person, although I was not an employee. Additionally, I was asked to commit to work at least three days each week to establish consistency with the clients. I agreed to these terms. Therefore, by the time I reported to Windy Hill on the first day of data collection, I was well acquainted with the basic structure and philosophy of Epworth. I had completed approximately 100 hours of observations and one-on-one training by the members of the corporate management team, in addition to having passed all physical and criminal examinations required of employees. Upon arrival at Windy Hill, I was

128

introduced as a staff person/intern. My three work days were Friday, Saturday and Monday which helped strengthen staff stability since the clients could depend upon my being there on the same days and at the same times each week. Data gathering was accomplished in several ways. I often wore a microphone so I could produce a running account of the day's activities and conversations. I always had my field notebook handy. In the early days I recorded notes directly into my 8 1/2" x 11" hardback field book; however, as I became more involved in the care of the clients, this was not practical, so I carried a smaller 3" x 6" pocket calendar and jotted notes that I later transcribed in detail in my field book. I was given access to the medical records of all clients. Documents, such as clients' notes to me or written directives for the day, were logged in the field book for later analysis. The monthly Rutledge Day Reviews were logged for analysis as well as some discussions with staff and family members of clients. Archival videotapes were made available, and I made notes in my field book of relevant data drawn from them.

The challenging level of organization required to keep two dozen clients and 8-10 staff members active for the 15 waking hours of each day first captured my attention. The organizational structure for each facility was based upon a traditional management hierarchy: facility manager, assistant managers, senior counselors, counselors. The day-to-day management of the activities was usually handled by one of the assistant managers because the manager was often engaged in addressing Epworth network responsibilities. The usual work week was 52 hours for full time employees. Most shifts were 10 hours long to provide continuity throughout the day for the clients. During the initial weeks of participation, my hours were generally 7:30 a.m. – 6:30 p.m. on Fridays; 8 a.m. – 3 p.m. on Saturdays, and 7:30 a.m. – 4 p.m. on Mondays. However, my involvement increased quickly as I saw avenues to pursue for my study. During the time of my study, we were often short staffed at Windy Hill, so the extra pair of hands seemed to be appreciated, and by October, my weekly schedule had increased from 30 to 40 hours. The log of my work schedule appears in Table 2

The main duty of a staff member was always the same: work side-by-side with the client in whatever activity he/she is attempting. During this shared work time, the goal of a staff member was not only to supervise and oversee the safety of the client, but also to serve as a role model for living by working side-by-side. The challenge, then, was to select the accurate "level" of a client's learning and engage him/her in successful steps from that point forward. As a staff member, I often caught myself feeling parental emotions, whether struggling to communicate with the lower-functioning client or attempting to redirect the higher-level client. The Epworth philosophy was that a productive person is a happy one, therefore, all daily activities were designed to be productive and never included work "invented" for the sake of work. Fortunately for me, the days selected provided me with a glimpse of the range and variety of activities in which clients were engaged. Because I predicted that the environmental context of this rehabilitation style might be critical to the motivational progress of each client, I will review the typical activities in which I was engaged while at work.

Friday: Clients' daily routines began at 6:30 a.m., with the exception of Sunday when they were able to sleep in until 7:00 a.m. Upon awaking, the client had time for a morning cup of coffee and a few moments with the daily newspaper if desired. Following this period, the client participated in morning stretches or walking exercises and a shower before breakfast. I generally arrived during breakfast. During breakfast, the assistant manager in charge would post a morning partner list outlining staff/client teams and their respective planned activities until lunch time. On Friday mornings, my early work assignment most often entailed working with clients on activities of daily living, called "ADLs" by the staff and clients, and overseeing the physical exercise routines for several clients while specifically assisting one or two who required one-on-one attention during exercises. This special attention was usually required due to a client's balance problems, poor concentration skills, or lack of understanding of the exercises. After the exercise session, which generally took about one hour, we enjoyed a coffee break before beginning morning academics. As each client's rehabilitation program was specifically designed just for him/her, so were the academics individually tailored. Often academic studies included, but were not limited to, exercises toward obtaining the GED (General Education Diploma), speech exercises, computer activities, letter writing, or reading. Academic exercises commanded the remainder of the morning activities. Other staff/client groups might engage in maintenance jobs around the facility, meal preparation, or arts and crafts instead of academic work. After lunch, everyone was involved in meal clean-up, including such chores as a complete washing of the floors, tables, and dishes, taking out the trash, and putting away any storable leftovers. Good personal hygiene was an important goal of Epworth's program, therefore emphasis was placed on brushing teeth after each meal.

Following this daily routine, the clients then entered their morning's activities in their journals. It was not uncommon first to have to assist the client in finding the journal before anything could be entered into it. Staff assisted the clients in journal entries, not by telling them what they had done but by cueing them to remember. One of the first things clients were encouraged to do is to keep a daily record of their activities in a small daily planner. The planners, similar to Franklin™ planners, were given to the clients monthly. Clients usually carried their planner, pens or other personal items they enjoyed having nearby (such as tissues) in a fanny pack.

Afternoon work projects followed until it was time for showers and dinner. The afternoon projects that were assigned included working in the garden tending to the vegetables, continuing facility maintenance jobs such as cutting the grass, picking pecans, washing the cars, cleaning the tool shed, raking the leaves, and typing simple office forms. Again, work breaks were given midway through the afternoon so no client ever felt "pushed" to work. By late afternoon the usual project for one staff/client team was the evening meal preparation. I was often assigned to assist with this. The menu was planned by the facility nutritionist and was prepared by the clients, under the supervision of staff. At Windy Hill, all clients were involved in meal preparation at one time or another, even though some were not allowed to work in the kitchen for safety reasons. Clients were taught how to organize kitchen duties as they worked side-by-side with the staff preparing the meal. Clients were not allowed, for safety reasons, to use the knives or cook with hot grease such as when preparing deep fried catfish. Usually on Friday evenings, I departed following the evening meal clean-up, prior to the beginning of group activities. On occasion, I stayed and assisted with special events such as the Halloween Dance or logged extra duty on the overnight shift.

Saturday: This was "adventure day" at Windy Hill as far as I was concerned. After staff/client partner assignments, all clients physically able to participate in the morning outing boarded the two vans and departed for the local high school track at 8:15 a.m. Able-bodied clients were required to walk the track four times (one mile). Those with ambulatory difficulties were encouraged to do as much as they could, and always to better their past time around the track. Staff were not excluded from this invigorating Saturday morning routine, but walked or jogged around the track depending upon the clients to whom they were assigned as partners for the morning. Having worked up quite an appetite, all then would head to a local favorite breakfast shop and spend the next hour enjoying the opportunity to be in the community "eating out like normal people." Breakfast orders were recorded by one staff member back at the facility in order to eliminate a bit of the confusion at the restaurant.

The final stop on the Saturday morning agenda was at one of the local washaterias. Imagine 20 people descending upon the washateria all at the same time, each with two to three loads of wash to be done! Each client was responsible for doing his/her own laundry, under the supervision of the staff. The staff spent a great deal of time teaching the details of how to do the wash. I quickly learned that while Saturday mornings were especially tiring physically and demanding mentally because we were in public and extra attention was needed for the clients, it was also a most rewarding teaching time. While washers were agitating and dryers spinning, precious captive minutes were available to the staff member just to chat and listen and guide the individuals.

The trip out on Saturday morning was often the highlight of the week for most of the clients at the Windy Hill program because they had not yet gained enough rank in the color categories to earn other outings. If a client had some sort of behavior problem at the facility, he/she was often put on "town restriction," meaning that he/she was not permitted to go on any group outing to town for 24 hours. Clients were particularly careful on Fridays, for they knew that Saturday's outing was just around the corner.

After all clothes were washed, dried and folded, clients returned to the facility for lunch. After the usual meal clean-up, teeth brushing and journal entry time, a thorough room cleaning and house cleaning would begin. Putting away all clean laundry and completely cleaning their rooms (including the bathrooms), sweeping and/or vacuuming the floors, cleaning windows, emptying trash, and straightening personal bookshelves were all on the client's Saturday afternoon schedule. After individual rooms were cleaned, the house (dorm) was cleaned with the same attention to detail. Staff again worked side-by-side with the clients as role models demonstrating proper ways to clean. The completion of cleaning was usually celebrated in the late afternoon with fruit or coffee prior to afternoon journal entries, showers, and dinner. Saturday evening activities included watching a video as a group or an outing of some sort. At the conclusion of each day, the clients met with staff to receive their "pay" for the day. Each time slot throughout the day was assigned a token money value (Table 5).

Table 5. Token Money Values

	All amounts are UP TO
Red & Orange Color Category	$5.00
TRACK	up to
STRETCH	$1.25
RUN	$2.50
BATH BFKST	$.50 each
CLEAN UP	$1.50
9-9:30 Annex	$2.50
A.M. WORK	$15.00
P: participation	$5.00
F: main focus	$5.00
A: attitude	$5.00
9:30 - 12:30	$15.00
JOURNAL	$1.25
BRUSHING	$.75
CHORE/SST	$2.50
P.M. WORK	$12.50
P: participation	$4.50
F: main focus	$4.00
A: attitude	$4.50
2:00 - 4:30	$12.50
SUBTOTAL	
RM/BATH	$.50 each
MEAL CLEAN	$2.00
ACTIVITY	$2.50
CLEAN UP	$1.50
S.S.T (social skills training) BONUS	$1.50
Daily Treatment Objective BONUS	$1.50

Clients were encouraged to recall their daily activities and were quizzed on the events of the day in an effort to increase their memory spans. Most of the clients at Windy Hill suffer with short term memory deficits.

Monday: On Mondays I was assigned often to be the staff member at the woodshop vocational work site. Departure time for work was between 8:45 and 9:00 a.m. As only certified staff were permitted to transport clients in the Epworth vehicles, careful planning was given to the coordination of work delivery. At the time of my internship four Windy Hill clients were employed at the woodshop. My responsibility at the woodshop most often included supervising all four of the Windy Hill woodshop employees because all were fairly self-sufficient at work. My responsibility, then, was to check clients' work periodically, be available to assist them when they became confused, and work alongside them in some assigned job that I was given by the woodshop manager. My assignments varied from the "stripping room" in which stripper was applied to furniture, to sanding furniture in preparation for staining, or assisting with the repair of antique furniture by holding parts with clients while epoxy set. Workers were given a break each hour during which time they gathered in the break room, and enjoyed interactions with clients from other Epworth network facilities. Because the Epworth network cares for well over 100 clients, the majority of whom work within one of the network vocational sites, staff and clients from all facilities can get to know one another. During the break, clients enjoyed a soda or Gatorade™ and snack, and entered their morning activities in their journals. Clients working in one of the Epworth facilities were taught to prepare their lunches the night before, so at lunch time they would once again gather in the break room to enjoy their sack lunches and fellow client socialization.

During the course of the morning's work, problems that might arise and require attention were both cognitive and behavioral in nature. For example, events that might create problems for a client were: sanding was not going fast enough, stripper solution was accidentally spilled on his/her shoes, or an angry reply was given when a client would forget for the third or fourth time the instructions of the morning. Clients working in the Epworth businesses had hours from 9:00 a.m. – 4:30 p.m. However, for Windy Hill clients on Mondays, the vocational work site day lasted only until noon. Clients returned to the facility for lunch.

Then, following meal clean-up, brushing teeth, and journal entries, they participated in the "arrangement meeting." For these meetings, the lunch tables were organized into a large 'conference table" and the clients gathered around the table to plan the coming week's activities. This procedure not only taught such organizational skills as personal planning and requesting permission for enacting such plans, but aided in social skills training, as each client had to listen to the others during the meeting. At Windy Hill, the arrangement meeting usually lasted two hours. Arrangements included such things as any snack items clients wished to purchase, telephone calls, shopping requests, or outing requests. Arrangements were recorded on a request sheet that the client could use to remember his/her desires during the meeting. Requests for any special privilege had to be submitted on a separate request sheet. Such privileges included a dinner outing with a staff member or family member, extra television privileges, karate lessons, shopping

137

trips, or attendance at AWARE (Always Wanted A Riding Experience). AWARE is the local equestrian club specializing in individuals with disabilities. The sheet had to be co-signed by the staff member to be involved, as well as the manager. During the arrangement meeting, token money awards were given to the client having the best journal entries for the previous week, the client earning the most money, and for extra jobs around the facility such as emptying all the wastebaskets regularly. Every effort was made to "catch the clients doing something right" and reward them. Following the arrangement meetings on Mondays, clients had their choice of activities such as traveling to the library, or working at the facility before the dinner hour. I usually left prior to dinner on Mondays.

My hours were fairly consistent during September. By October my involvement with the clients and stresses engendered by staffing shortages, caused me voluntarily to increase my hours by almost three each day; therefore, by mid-October I was averaging 40 hours per week at the Windy Hill facility. My period for Rotation 1 ended November 8, 1997. During the following week (November 9 – November 15, 1997), I participated in the Brain Injury Education Program for Certified Brain Injury Specialists.

ROTATION 2

Rotation 2 began on November 17, 1997 at the Tallangatta facility, the community reentry program. The Tallangatta program was the top level of the multi-level Epworth Rehabilitation Network. Clients living at this facility had the highest level functioning, physically, mentally, emotionally, and behaviorally of all Epworth clients. Residents in this program lived either in one of the group homes, or in apartments. While the basic philosophy of the Epworth structure was followed at all facilities, the Tallangatta program allowed the most "freedom" of daily activities for each individual client. Transfer criteria from any of the primary facilities to the Tallangatta program required that the client had successfully negotiated five levels in the color category strategy. Once "promoted" to the Tallangatta program, the client was allowed to earn U.S. currency and apply for a community job or continue at the site of their network vocational job. Some of the Tallangatta residents were full-time students in the local university or high schools. My schedule at the Tallangatta program was the same as the regular, full-time staff, 52 hours per week. My usual work days were from Friday – Monday. Because my "work week" span was only four days not five, Fridays and Mondays were usually 12-hour shifts, 7:30 a.m. – 7:30 p.m.. Saturdays and Sundays were generally 14-hour shifts, 8 a.m. – 10 p.m. In the weeks during my university Christmas break, I spent extra hours at the Tallangatta program. My work log appears in Table 2.

Because one of the requirements for residency at the Tallangatta program was a full-time job, either at network-owned or community-based, no clients were "home" during the day, unless, of course, they had worked during the night before, or they were ill. The primary function of the community reentry program was to prepare the client for life in the community. All activities, such as weekly blood tests, vocational testing, personal desires such as trips to Wal-Mart™, etc. had to be planned for by the client around his/her work schedule, just as would be done in the "real world." Because the focus of the Tallangatta program is community reentry, staff responsibilities were different than those at the primary facilities, where the focus centered around the basics of proper behavior and skills such as memory and sequencing. While the Epworth philosophy was implemented in the Tallangatta program, two major differences were the money system and staff supervision. Like all other programs, the staff were given their partner lists for activities. Unlike in the other programs, Tallangatta staff were role-modeling cognitive strategies for daily living more than behavioral coping skills. Care was given to provide each individual with a personalized schedule within the structure.

The Tallangatta program was located in the heart of the small community, thus making many places of interest for the upper-level client within walking distance. The residency at Tallangatta fluctuated between two and three dozen, with the ratio of men to women again being consistent (4-1) with national percentages. At Tallangatta, work week activities centered around the client's job. Personal responsibilities such as grocery shopping or laundry had to be addressed on the weekend. Clients in the Tallangatta program were not all herded in one large group to outings as they were at the primary facilities; they went in smaller groups. Personal chores often separated men from women. Each week was a bit different in the hourly structure and organization in Tallangatta, just as it would be for us in "real life"; therefore, I will offer a sample of my work schedule.

Friday and Monday: Unlike my staff introductions at the Windy Hill program, I was just "thrown in" to work, with no real introduction to clients. I explained that I was a student intern and had just been transferred from Windy

Hill. Because the Epworth facilities work so closely together, I already knew many of the clients. A typical Friday and Monday for me often included the woodshop work run. I usually arrived during breakfast time. Following breakfast, clients followed the same routine as at Windy Hill, including meal clean-up, brushing teeth then preparing to leave for work. For me and those clients who were not reporting to an outside job, the first hour and a half was spent at another network facility exercise room, with the Tallangatta clients each following their personalized exercise routines. Staff members were assigned to several clients and, like at other facilities, were to work alongside the client. Following the exercise program, I went to the woodshop with my partners for the duration of the day. My responsibilities during this time were identical to those described during my Windy Hill days at the woodshop. Being assigned to the woodshop gave me the opportunity to continue to follow the progress of my Windy Hill clients while getting to know my Tallangatta clients.

Evening activities at the Tallangatta program basically followed the general Epworth structure: journal entries, meal prep, meal clean-up, and brushing teeth. Clients in the Tallangatta program used the time in the evenings to prepare for work the next day by preparing their lunch and checking clothes. On Friday evenings in Tallangatta, usually the women would go to the washateria while the men would engage in some group activity such as watching a video after all inventory had been completed for the Saturday shopping chores. Monday evenings were devoted to the Tallangatta arrangement meetings. Unlike at the primary facilities, where arrangements were held as a group affair, individuals in the Tallangatta program met independently with the assistant managers to get

141

approval on their arrangements for the week. In addition to their arrangement meeting, the Tallangatta clients had to meet with their banking partner to account for their money for the week. Each Tallangatta client had the opportunity to open a bank account in the community, with a staff co-signature. It was a goal for clients that they learn to write checks, budget their finances, and be accountable for money. Privileges were revoked if the client did not exercise good financial judgment. When this happened, the client was given the opportunity to regain his/her account by earning back the right, in the same way he/she gained it in the first place.

Saturday: For the working person, Saturdays are full days. For the client in Tallangatta it was no different. Following a leisurely Saturday morning breakfast, the clients separated to take care of personal responsibilities. Often my assignment was to accompany the men during the day. The morning chore was often a trip to the washateria and in the afternoon, we took a trip to the grocery store. Unlike the clients at the primary facilities, the clients at the Tallangatta program did their own individual shopping, divided into three sections: meal preparation, inventory, and personal. The client shopped for the food needed for the meal he/she was assigned to prepare for the week, then he/she gathered the items for the facility pantry from his/her inventory section, and finally he/she gathered his/her personal goods. The grocery list was approved prior to departure for the grocery store and initialed by one of the assistant managers. The client was then responsible for his/her own money to pay for his/her personal items. The items for his/her meal preparation and the general inventory were transferred to the staff at the check-out and the Epworth network paid for these items. The afternoons were filled with putting away the groceries purchased, cleaning rooms, house, and grounds, then usually relaxing and enjoying television. On Saturday evenings, clients would go in all directions on outings, such as the movies or dinner out, joining the group video session, or just having personal time.

Sunday: Sunday activities were largely focused around a day of rest and relaxation for the clients. Morning responsibilities for the staff usually fell into one of two categories: a church outing or academics. I had the opportunity to participate in both activities. One of the joys was being assigned to attend church. Because these clients were high functioning and needed very little assistance in community settings, church was a pleasant and relaxing outing. For those clients not attending church, academic time was scheduled in the classroom to work on their individual programs. For those clients attending the local high school or university, there was always homework to be done. Academics at the Tallangatta program were similar to those of the Windy Hill program with the exception that the clients were at a higher-functioning level. Often on Sundays after the group returned from church, all would head for lunch out and a movie in town as a group. The role of the staff members during these outings was to assist the clients in the finer skills needed socially, or to think through situations and learn how to problem solve. The challenge for the staff at this level was to understand a bit about how individuals learn and to be able to offer constructive cognitive strategies. Sunday evenings usually included quiet activities back at the program as the clients prepared for the coming work week.

My two months at the Tallangatta program were completed on January 12, 1998. The data gathering in Tallangatta differed from that of the Windy Hill program, as clients were anxious to share their opinions but preferred not being recorded throughout the day. I quickly became a comrade when they discovered that I, too, had suffered a brain injury. Often the clients wanted to discuss personal topics "off the record." Therefore, I relied on my calendar pocketbook for recording notes critical to my research, which I then transcribed into my field book. The other documentation such as medical records, archival video, and Rutledge Review days, notes, etc. was available to me at this site as it was at Windy Hill. Interviews were conducted with the Tallangatta clients, and these were audiorecorded. Following my full-time involvement at the site, I continued throughout the spring to work one day a week as a staff member in order to follow the progress and sustained motivation of my participating clients.

Data: Collection and Analysis Process

Doing qualitative research, for me, was like accepting the challenge to work a jigsaw puzzle with no identification of the picture to emerge. Having accepted this challenge, I learned that not only did I not have an image of the final picture but I didn't have any of the puzzle pieces or shapes which I had to find before I could begin to assemble the picture of my findings. The rewards of qualitative research come in seeing the "picture" evolve as you find one puzzle piece at a time, analyze it, match it, or discard it, then look for the next piece.

In this type of research, data collection and analyses are not two distinct processes; rather they are intertwined and studied in a recursive fashion. Data are analyzed as they are collected, and this analysis guides the researcher toward further data collection, which, in turn, directs the investigator toward more refined and focused data collection and analysis as the project unfolds.

To facilitate the emergent process of this research design, I was attentive to the early needs of planning. Needs included negotiating and developing conditions for entry into my sites, the logistics of how and what data would be collected to ensure trustworthiness, purposive sampling, and design (Erlandson, Harris, Skipper & Allen, 1993, p. 69). I began data collection with a set of observation guidelines in mind such as:

- How would I describe the facilities?
- How would I describe the clientele?
- How are the rehabilitation programs planned for each client?
- Are the clients' injuries similar?
- Are there common problems of behavior? Cognitive challenges?
- How would I describe the staff?
- How do the staff respond to clients? To other staffers? To families? To me?
- What is the paperwork trail? How is it related to each client on a daily basis?
- What is the morale of the clients?

As discussed earlier, during the first several weeks I was involved in training and observation. During these days my entries into my field book were on the nature of questions I wanted to remember to ask, or events I saw and wanted to explore, or relationships I wished to pursue. These entries were made in addition to notations of what I was observing. During the early weeks,

145

following each day's activities, I would audiotape my feelings and thoughts on my 45-minute drive home. Once home, before returning to the facility, for the next data collection session, I listened to the tape and made additional notes. As the weeks stretched into months, this plan was abandoned for two reasons: I was gathering plenty of data via audiotape and journal entries during the day, and I was simply exhausted on the trip home and needed to concentrate on driving.

At the end of each week of participation I submitted the audiotapes to my transcriptionist. Within a fortnight she delivered each set of text files, which enabled me to begin coding the data and formulating refinements to the process. The analysis of qualitative data is an ongoing process, not an after-the-fact event. The analysis actually began the first day I arrived on site. As cited in Erlandson, Harris, Skipper & Allen (1993, p. 111) Marshall and Rossman explain:

> Data analysis is the process of bringing order, structure, and meaning to the mass of collected data. It is a messy, ambiguous, time-consuming, creative, and fascinating process. It does not proceed in a linear fashion; it is not neat. Qualitative data analysis is a search for general statements about relationship among categories of data; it builds grounded theory. (p. 111)

As noted earlier, multiple conversations and interviews, as well as archival data such as videos, documents, records were audiotaped and/or entered into the field books. I followed the coding procedures recommended by Strauss and Corbin (1990). Often grounded theory is referred to as "the constant comparative method of analysis" (Glaser & Strauss, 1967, pp. 101-116) because analytic procedure is closely related to the strategy for doing research, which has the same name. During data analysis, the first analytic function is to make a comparison of data, and the second procedure is to ask questions pertaining to that data.

The first process I performed on my raw data was to conceptualize what I had recorded. I systematically took apart conversations, events, dialogue, incidents, ideas shared, and events that occurred by marking in the margins of the transcript sections I felt had any kind of message for motivation. Next, I gave each idea a label. The 210 different conceptual labels are in Appendix E. Examples of label names are distrust, being watched, goals, fear of the outside, money, proof, uncomfortable, obsession, humor, control, limits, learn by rote, timing, opinion, rewards, mistakes, solitude, Bible, outing, ZPD, staff tips, etc. This process of assigning labels to "chunks" of data is called open coding (Strauss and Corbin, 1990). At the conclusion of each coding session, I wrote big new labels created on white board space (3 ft. x 8 ft.) in my office. As the days passed, I began the "comparative" (Strauss and Corbin, 1990) step by determining common properties of concepts, thus creating categories. As I noted several that looked similar, I would rearrange them on the white board into a category. As I located matching items in the data to labels already on the board, the page reference in the transcriptions would be noted on the board. For example, for a reference to the Bible, I might enter "3, F75, 84, 450, D1." That code signalled to me that in the transcriptions notations appear on pages 3, 84, and 450; reference was made to the Bible in my field book on page 75 and in document 1. Often at this stage, I used Post-it-Notes™ to enter ideas near categories until it was clear that these ideas belonged in the same category. On the other side of my office, a large pegboard (4 ft. x 8 ft.) held not only categorized journal articles from my review of literature but also documents and artifacts from the research site that I wanted to study. Often these documents were shuffled from one peg to another,

147

grouping them in a similar manner to the labels from the transcriptions. As a major category would emerge from studying the documents, the label would be transferred to the whiteboard. Truly, this experience was that of the end product being the revised revision of the original revised revision revised.

During the categorizing phase of analysis, I would ask questions when in the field that would assist me in building the dimensions or properties of each category identified (Strauss & Corbin, 1990). The emerging categories were abstracted units that contained subcategories, resulting from my open coding process. Ultimately, these categories became the conceptual units from which the theory emerged. As encouraged by Strauss and Corbin (1990), I used code notes (labels I assigned), theoretical notes (notes to myself of questions generated from my code notes), and operational notes (directions to myself for further investigation) to assist in this data analysis process. I made every attempt to be attentive to the need to enhance my theoretical sensitivity through comparisons, questions, listening, and observing.

Concurrent to the activities of coding the transcriptions of data, I was returning to the field for 40 hours each week, building upon the impressions I was seeing emerge on my whiteboard at the same time I was observing and experiencing new data. The second phase of my analysis was that of axial coding. Strauss and Corbin (1990) described axial coding as the process of reconstructing categories to make connections and relationships between categories and their subcategories. The goal in this stage of coding is to specify a category in terms of its conditions; that is, the context in which it is embedded, the interactional strategies by which it is carried out, and the consequences of those strategies.

(Strauss & Corbin, 1990, p. 97-115). During the beginning stages of this coding segment, I used 5" x 8" note cards on which to record ideas and test relationships among data. Sitting before my whiteboards, I would return to the transcript and jot down key ideas from the labels created for specific data categories. Then I would do the same for another label on the whiteboard that I thought might link to the one I had just revised. After repeating this procedure for days and weeks, refining data analysis by asking additional questions in the field or seeking additional forms of data, I was able to create major theme categories from these labels. For example, I was able to link subcategories such as "anger, staff time, limits, money, and control" together to form a relationship that resulted in the category called, "Demotivators." These categories are called contextual categories (Strauss and Corbin, 1990).

As quoted from Marshall and Rossman (in Erlandson, Harris, Skipper, & Allen, 1993), analysis "does not proceed in a linear fashion..." (p. 112). Therefore, during the cyclical processes of open and axial coding, I was continuing to return to the field, gather additional data, refine the emerging themes, and return home to begin the process all over again in analysis, building each time upon the latest interpretation as my findings were emerging.

Selective coding was the third type of data analysis used in this study. This coding method helped to relate notions of motivation to the categories that emerged, and to interpret and validate these relationships. This confounding task is the gateway to the formation of the researcher's grounded theory model. Integrating all the various categories, studying them again in light of salient properties, dimensions, and paradigmatic relationships is challenging. There are

149

several steps to selective coding, according to Strauss and Corbin (1990): explicate a story line, relate subsidiary categories around the core category, relate categories at dimensional levels, validate the previous steps, and finally, look for any weak spots and fill in with further refinement through field work. What emerges from these selective coding processes is simply a descriptive overview of the findings. In developing this story line, I used the 1 1/2-hour travel time each day to reflect upon my months of research experience, imagining myself standing before an audience to describe my experiences. As I "spoke" to these various imaginary audiences I had created in my mind, I discovered that though perhaps phrased slightly different to attend to audience needs, I was beginning to tell the same story to each "audience."

The core category began to emerge at this point (Strauss and Corbin, 1990). As the weeks passed, I kept my different "speech ideas" posted on my pegboard so that they remained constantly in front of me. When an idea no longer appeared regularly in my imaginary "speeches" delivered in the car during my travel time, it was removed from the list, and others were added. Finally, these imaginary "speeches" (of course, all delivered to enthusiastic audiences!) were then reduced into short stories that could convey the motivational factors influencing individuals with TBI in their recovery.

Although these steps have been discussed in a linear manner, it needs to be noted that these processes were not linear, but rather were more parallel in nature. As investigators, we like to think of grounded theory as a transactional system (Strauss and Corbin, 1990), a method of analysis that allows us to examine the interactive nature of events. Once the basics of coding have been completed, a researcher is able to create a framework, called the conditional matrix (Strauss and Corbin, 1990), that enables the researcher to distinguish and link levels of conditions and consequences. This matrix helped me to begin to draw conclusions about factors that were similarly expressed in all TBI clients, rather than isolating them specifically according to the nature of their injuries. Throughout the process, I endeavored periodically to sample and test the emerging theories by observing them from all viewpoints available to me, and by checking my ideas with all participants, including those in the preliminary studies.

In order to validate the outcomes of my coding and categories, I enlisted the assistance of three judges: my colleague Dr. Barbara Holmes, the Clinical Director for the Epworth Rehabilitation Network, and Jeanne Moore, Neurorehabilitation Specialist at the University of Texas Southwestern Medical Center at Dallas. First, after coding and categorizing nearly all the data I shared the raw data, and my coding categories with Barbara. She read the data, then my notes and categories. She then made a judgment as to whether she felt the data coding was accurate or not. Barbara evaluated the majority of the raw data in this manner. We agreed on every category I had entered and there were no discrepancies between us. Her input was aided by the fact that she had completed a visit to the facility, observing my work with the clients. She did offer several suggestions for further consideration of subcategories.

Second, after creating the draft of my grounded theory model, I met with the Clinical Director of Epworth and shared the model with him. I presented the model and supported my reasons for its design based upon what I had observed at the facilities. He was in total agreement with my ideas, stating more than once

151

that he was pleased that I seemed to have captured the very "essence of Epworth."
He also stated that he felt that the model graphically illustrated his thoughts about
triggers of motivation. He also offered two further areas to consider for inclusion
in the model which were based upon trends he had observed over the years. I
returned to the data to assess his ideas, and did find the trends he mentioned.
Therefore, they, too, were incorporated into my findings.

Finally, I sought to validate the final model by seeking the opinion of a
neurorehabilitation specialist, Jeanne Moore. Jeanne's years of experience with
neurological patients at the University of Texas Southwestern Medical Center at
Dallas offered the insight of a medical practitioner to the results. I was pleased
that Jeanne found the model that emerged to be one of "workable potential" for
her patients. She shared concerns of the effects "too much support" may have on
momentum, a consideration we decided deserved attention in future studies. An
interesting insight offered by Jeanne was that of the teaching potential for staff
through the model.

Summary

"Every research study, qualitative or quantitative, must be evaluated in
terms of the specific canons and procedures of the research method that was used
to generate the findings" (Strauss & Corbin, 1990, p. 258). In this chapter, I have
outlined the methods chosen for this study as well as the evaluative procedures
undertaken to ensure its trustworthiness and authenticity. In addition to the
methodological discussion, I sought to offer a "thick description" of the events of

my field activity, data collection, and data analysis. Strauss and Corbin (1990, p. 259) cite John Dewey at the conclusion of their grounded theory text. I find the citation a fitting transition to Chapter 5, a discussion of my "work:"

"It is no linguistic accident that 'building,' 'construction,' 'work,' designate both a process and its finished product. Without the meaning of the verb that of the noun remains blank." (Dewey, 1934, p. 51)

CHAPTER 5

"Like an arc. Say you have an arc and you're figuring the degrees of the arc by measuring the amount of the angles and you find out how the arc works. But that doesn't work any more, so you're saying, 'okay, I'll do something else.' And you figure out how this arc works, too. But, those arcs will never intersect. So, I was always trying, I've been trying to intersect the arcs that will not intersect."

-Ray, Tallangatta client

Introduction

With eloquence, Ray defined the frustrations that come from the efforts of an individual struggling in traumatic brain injury (TBI) rehabilitation. An individual with TBI may feel his/her life has been shattered and jumbled, much as the kaleidoscope that has been broken and no longer yields geometrically balanced and beautiful designs in a prism of colors, arcs that will no longer intersect but come ever so close. Whether expressed openly or unexpressed and held silently within, each individual lives by a set of norms and values for his/her life; therefore, our perceptions of life vary one from another. These individual perceptions are disrupted when an individual suffers TBI.

As simple as it looks, the kaleidoscope yields the most complex geometric designs; likewise, the simple word *motivation* is merely the shell for a complex set of relationships found in this study. I had considered presenting "motivation" by a clear, simple definition followed by examples of the manifestations of the various *motivational theories* I had studied: intrinsic, extrinsic, disengagement, psychological/cognitive/emotional, transtheoretical, or self-determination, to name a few. While, the complexity of this phenomenon defied discussion at that simple categorized level, the data gathered did yield a common bond among those in rehabilitation: *momentum*. Whether this momentum was firmly established and strong enough to propel the volitional qualities of an individual over time, then, was the elusive *motivation* I sought to define.

To assist in the comprehension of the complex relationships discovered, I will present these findings in the following manner. To offer the reader insights into the multifaceted personal factors bearing influence upon the momentum of an individual with TBI, I will introduce eight composite individuals (six clients, two staff) in a case study format. Following these composite introductions, a brief discussion of the study's outcomes and consequences is presented in order to highlight the relationship of the contextual categories to the central phenomenon. Finally, each contextual category is presented concluding with a discussion of the interactional strategies and illustrated by particular examples from the data. All quotes are direct transcriptions reflecting how individuals stated them, and are not necessarily grammatically correct.

PARTICIPANT COMPOSITES

One of the strengths of qualitative study is the richness of detail that can be obtained from observing and or participating in a particular phenomenon and the interactions within that phenomenon. While this wealth of detail is a strength, it can also confound the researcher attempting to capture the essence of the interactions in mere words. To create a participant description of each client actively involved in this study not only would entail many pages, but also would not necessarily aid in the readers' understanding of the momentum of motivation,

155

the heart of this study. Therefore, after wrestling with the dilemma of creating a vicarious experience of introduction to these participants, I have chosen to create six composite individuals. These individuals represented three types of clients with whom I worked during each rotation.

First, I will introduce Frances and Kellan, to represent the many short-term clients at the Windy Hill and Tallangatta programs respectively. Frances and Kellan, and clients like them, were sent to Epworth by one of several agencies funding short-term rehabilitation services. Their stay would be between three and six months with possible, but not necessarily probable, extensions. Next, I present Larry of Windy Hill and Kenneth of Tallangatta . These two young men are similar to the clients with unlimited funding and, at this point, uncertain futures. Both are hopeful of ultimately living within their communities again. Finally, I will present Ricardo and Danica, again clients of Windy Hill and Tallangatta respectively. These two composites represent the lifelong clients at Epworth, not capable of living independently, but, in a group-home, able to enjoy productive lives in supported community living situations. All six of these TBI clients are composite profiles of several matching categories, not a representation of any single individual.

Staff interactions are critical to the momentum of TBI client. In addition to the clients, I will offer two staff composites. I worked with over 34 staff members, 14 closely. Over the months of observing client/staff interactions, personal interactions, and client reactions, I noted characteristics of staff members, some of which made them effective, others less effective. The characteristics of the effective staff member are illustrated in the composite staff member, Colton Criswell. The negative traits and characteristics are embodied in the character of Anna Ratchett. Fortunately, most of the staff members with whom I worked are positive and Anna Ratchett represents only one in every five staffers.

These composite descriptions, both client and staff, are intended for illustrative purposes only. Later in this chapter, wherever transcriptions appear, the word "snip" designates dialogue that has been omitted.

FRANCES: SHORT-TERM WINDY HILL COMPOSITE CLIENT

History Prior to the Injury: Frances was a 22-year-old single, white female. She was the youngest of three children. Her parents lived in the small town where Frances grew up, about 400 miles from the rehabilitation facility. Frances was a high school cheerleader and was active in many school clubs such as Future Homemakers and the debate team. Her grades reflected her heavy extracurricular activities; however, she was a solid 'B' student. Following high school graduation, Frances entered the local community college and was a sophomore at the time of the accident. Frances continued to be active in the community, volunteering at the local nursing home and working at the Hamburger Hangout on the week-ends. Church activities also consumed much of her time.

Family History: Frances's father was a long-distance trucker, who was often away from home for long periods of time; however, he was most supportive and anxious to provide for the family in every way. Frances's mother was a homecare

157

nursing assistant sitting with the elderly. At the time of this study, both of the older siblings of this composite client were married and living away from home. Frances was living in an apartment with three friends at the time of the accident. Immediately following the accident, Frances's father secured the power of attorney as well as guardianship over his daughter's financial and personal affairs.

Injury History: Approximately 14 months ago, Frances was an unrestrained back seat passenger in a small car driven by one of her roommates. Frances was thrown from the car when it was rear-ended by a pick-up truck; she suffered a dislocated left shoulder, compound-complex fracture of the left tibula/fibula and multiple bruises and lacerations. Secondary to the accident, Frances suffered a traumatic brain injury to her left frontal and temporal lobes as well as damage to the motor-cortex. Frances was unconscious for 11 days and had a post-traumatic amnesia of about 24 days. After her release from the hospital, Frances was taken home for care and outpatient rehabilitation at the local hospital. During these day sessions in rehabilitation, Frances had right-sided upper and lower hemiparesis, as well as Broca's aphasia. Frances had late onset seizures at nine months post-injury.

Current Physical and Medical Condition: At the time of this study, Frances was 24 years old, 5 feet 7 inches tall, and weighed 150 pounds. She had a basilar skull fracture and cerebellar damage that contributed to her ataxia. She had hearing loss in the left ear at low frequency. She continued to have right-sided hemiparesis which required her to use a cane. Her gait was most unsteady. Her medication was Tegretol and Folic acid to prevent distortions of the red blood cells. Frances had gained 30 pounds since her accident and was not receptive to physical exercises. This was attributed to lack of initiative stemming from the frontal lobe injury.

Current Cognitive Status: The primary deficits in cognitive functioning for this composite client, Frances, were communication problems. Since she had mild Broca's aphasia, she struggled with complex messages or instructions. She had great difficulty in routine activities of daily living (ADLs) especially showering. Her short-term memory was weak.

Current Behavioral Status: Because her gait was unsteady, she wore a gait belt with on-hands assist. She had to be supervised at all times to keep her safe. She became agitated when confused and would curse and yell in a loud voice. She was occasionally non-compliant, but usually would take direction. Frances was quiet and shy unless agitated. Frances liked chewing gum, coffee, snacks of all kinds, and personal attention.

Funding and Discharge Options: Like many short-term clients, Frances was funded by the state branch of the federal rehabilitation commission and had been assigned a personal rehabilitation counselor by the commission. The initial funding was for three months with a three-month extension available, if merited. The family hoped to have Frances return home, be employable at a low-functioning community job, and be able to achieve some independence in life,

159

either in a nearby group home for brain-injured individuals, or perhaps in the additional wing they had attached to their home. The group home to which they were referred cared for individuals of many types of brain injury or disorder, for example: all gradations of retardation, Down's Syndrome, cerebral palsy, multiple sclerosis, and stroke.

KELLAN: SHORT-TERM TALLANGATTA COMPOSITE CLIENT

History Prior to the Injury: Kellan was a 33-year-old white male. He was the eldest of two children. His birth father and mother were divorced, and the younger sibling resided with the birth mother. Kellan was reared by relatives since his parents could not afford to care for him in the early days. He was a high achiever throughout school and was in the senior year at a large university at the time of his accident 14 years ago. In high school, he focused on graphic arts. He was not much of a sportsman. In college, he preferred books to people, describing himself as a "nerd." At the time of his accident, he was single and has remained so.

Family History: Kellan had no relationship with his father and appeared to be very close to his foster mother. His younger brother, 22, was in his final year of university at the time of this study. The brother had been attentive to Kellan in the last several years. However, in the early years post-injury, friction existed between the two. The foster father had been an itinerant mechanic while Kellan was growing up, so they moved frequently, thus Kellan had no "roots" in any particular place. His foster parents had moved several times since his accident.

Injury History: Kellan was an unrestrained passenger thrown from the bed of a pick-up truck. He suffered multiple abrasions of his lower extremities as well as fractures to his left foot and right femur. His CT scan revealed diffuse cerebral hemorrhaging with basilar skull fracture. He was comatose for five days and suffered post-traumatic amnesia for 23 days. He had some left-ear hearing loss. Kellan had had five dental surgeries, all accident related, at the time of this study.

Current Physical and Medical Condition: Kellan lost 50 pounds during the months of dental surgeries due to having his mouth wired closed. He weighed 176 pounds and stood 6 feet 4 inches tall at the time of this study. He fatigued easily and had no stamina. He was on no medications and had no seizure history.

Current Cognitive Status: Kellan was distracted easily, had poor short-term memory, social skills, judgment, and problem-solving skills. He exhibited quick temper outbursts and frustration resulting in mood swings. His insight into his deficits was poor.

Current Behavioral Status: Other than the emotional outbursts, Kellan's behavior was fairly stable. He tended to be impulsive around food and, at times, could be socially inappropriate around women.

Funding and Discharge Options: Kellan was funded through the state branch of the federal rehabilitation commission. A six-month treatment time had been granted with only vocational extensions possible. His family had requested that his short-term memory be improved and that Kellan be able to live independently upon return to the community.

LARRY: OUTCOME UNKNOWN WINDY HILL COMPOSITE CLIENT

History Prior to the Injury: Larry was a lethargic 19-year-old white male. He was the youngest of two children. His father and mother resided in a distant state. Larry was an under-achiever academically in high school. While he had been popular in school largely due to his athletic abilities and winsome personality, he was a drifter after high school. At the time of his accident he had been a part-time worker at three fast-food restaurants, an automotive service station, and a delivery service. He had no ability to remain in a job.

Family History: Even though Larry's family resided in a distant state, they visited frequently. At the time of this study, this composite client's older sister was married and living in a neighboring state and also often visited. At the time of my interview with Larry, his parents were still his legal guardians as well as holders of his power of attorney. The family was supportive as were a large circle of friends and relatives.

Injury History: Larry was thrown from his bicycle when brushed by a mirror on the side of a delivery truck. His bike helmet was jarred from his head, and his head hit a curb causing a subdural hematoma in the left temporal lobe of the brain. Larry was anoxic for several minutes until revived. He was unconscious for 11 days. Post-traumatic amnesia lasted approximately 35 days. Larry was hospitalized at the trauma center for four weeks, then transferred to the rehabilitation branch of the hospital. Larry exhibited some right-sided upper and lower extremity hemiparesis and moderate Wernicke's aphasia while in the rehabilitation center. He was disoriented and had a poor short-term memory. He remained an outpatient for six months prior to attempting academic reentry. His initial attempts at academic work were unsuccessful.

Current Physical and Medical Condition: At the time of the study Larry was 6 feet tall and weighed 215 pounds. He wore contacts to correct visual acuity. He had had no episodes of seizures. He was currently on no medications. The right-sided hemiparesis had diminished and was only prevalent when he was fatigued.

Current Cognitive Status: Larry appeared to have no residual effects of the Wernicke's aphasia; however, he became confused rather easily as a result of his inability to sequence. He had difficulty in remaining focused on tasks and tended to perseverate on past events.

Current Behavioral Status: Larry's emotional stability was the prime concern. He enjoyed physical workouts, sports of all kinds, and snack foods, especially M & M's.

Funding and Discharge Options: The funding for Larry was provided through the group insurance of the delivery company. Ultimately, Larry wanted to resume independent living and his college matriculation.

KENNETH: OUTCOME UNKNOWN TALLANGATTA COMPOSITE CLIENT

History Prior to the Injury: Kenneth was a 34-year-old white male. He was married and the father of two children. Kenneth was a solid student in high school and college. In high school, he participated in extra-curricular activities such as sports, drama, and service clubs. He was elected "Most Likely to Succeed" his senior year. During college, he played football while earning a degree in business. Up until his accident, he was an accountant for a large firm. He and his wife had been married for 14 years. This composite client had a 12-year-old daughter, and a 6-year-old son at the time of this study. Kenneth and his family were active in church and community affairs. Therefore, he had a large support structure including family, friends, work associates, and community contacts.

Family History: Kenneth's parents lived in the same community as Kenneth and his wife. They had moved in with the daughter-in-law in order to assist with the household responsibilities in Kenneth's absence.

Injury History: Kenneth was a restrained passenger in a car that was hit head on by an out-of-control 14-ton flat-bed truck. Kenneth suffered multiple fractures to his back, jaw, sternum, pelvis, and right foot. The coup-contracoup injury immediately rendered Kenneth unconscious. His heart stopped at the scene, and he was anoxic for several minutes until revived. The CT scan taken at the trauma hospital showed a transverse skull fracture from the base to the front and a subdural hematoma near the left lobes of the brain. Though never in a deep comatose state, Kenneth drifted in and out of consciousness for 5 days following the accident and experienced post-traumatic amnesia for approximately 32 days. Kenneth required no surgery for fractures, but did require months of confinement to bed in addition to a cervical orthotic device to stabilize his thoraco-cervical spine and support his head. Kenneth was transferred following hospitalization to an outpatient status for rehabilitation. Following late onset post-traumatic grand-mal seizures, he was readmitted to the hospital for a period of four months during which time he received extensive speech, physical, and cognitive therapy while the seizures were being monitored and brought under medicated control. Kenneth was disoriented and easily agitated. His short-term memory was poor, and his long-term memory was patchy. He exhibited some problems with speech, especially stuttering.

Current Physical and Medical Condition: Kenneth was in excellent health and had seizures under control at the time of the study. He was on Tegretol and Elavil, dosages unknown. He enjoyed exercise, sports, especially golfing. Kenneth was 6 feet tall and weighed 220 pounds. He had hearing loss to high frequency sounds.

Current Cognitive Status: Kenneth's deficits were both communicative and organizational in nature. He comprehended information, yet had trouble processing answers quickly. His math skills seemed to be intact, though weak at this point. Kenneth had great difficulty in organizational skills. His attention span was short.

Current Behavioral Status: Kenneth could follow instructions and worked independently quite well until he became confused. Confusion triggered his temper and outbursts could be volatile. Kenneth had extreme difficulty in problem-solving and executive skills, such as planning, and decision making. He liked M & M's , Dr. Pepper, and bananas. He did not drink coffee.

Funding and Discharge Options: Kenneth was funded by private insurance.

RICARDO: LIFE RESIDENT WINDY HILL COMPOSITE CLIENT

History Prior to the Injury: At the time of his accident, Ricardo was a 52-year-old Hispanic, married and the father of four. He was the youngest of eight children. Both parents were deceased. Ricardo was a migrant farm worker throughout his early school years. He attended a mid-sized university on a migrant scholarship program; however, he dropped out after struggling academically. Ricardo married for the first time at age 25. Two children were born, but this marriage ended in divorce after eight years. Ricardo was married again for a short period in his late thirties. No children were born during this marriage. Following his second wife's death, Ricardo began to drink heavily. After receiving an honorable discharge from an alcohol rehabilitation facility, Ricardo joined a local security company serving shopping centers. Ricardo married for a third time at the age of 48. He had two children from this marriage, a daughter, eighteen months and a son, three years old at the time of the accident.

Family History: Ricardo's parents were deceased. He was widowed by his second wife and his first wife still resided in the town. While he did not have opportunity to see his siblings often, the two eldest sisters and the brother just older than Ricardo had been most attentive since the accident. His children by his first wife rushed to his bedside affirming their concern for his recovery and offering their attention to handling his business matters. This gesture was greeted with animosity from the current wife as well as his siblings. Neither of his children had spoken to his third wife in the previous eight years. Though a tangled web to understand, this composite client appeared to have a broad base of support.

Injury History: While on security duty 11 years ago, Ricardo was answering a store robbery call that suddenly erupted into gunfire. Ricardo was wounded in the right frontal region of his brain. The bullet traversed the brain from the right to its exit in the left occipital region. Ricardo was comatose for three weeks. Post-traumatic amnesia was approximately 23 days. Following six weeks of hospitalization, Ricardo was transferred to a nursing home for care where he had remained for eight years with no aggressive rehabilitation program until admission to Windy Hill.

Current Physical and Medical Condition: Ricardo had upper left extremity hemiplegia. He was ambulatory on a quad cane, having been out of a wheelchair for five weeks. Speech was slow, slurred, and weak. He continued to experience some visual difficulties and a need for glasses was indicated.

Current Cognitive Status: Ricardo appeared to be mentally dull with moments of lucidity. Short-term memory was weak. Sequencing was difficult for Ricardo when he was tired. Learning was from role modeling, rather than from visual memory.

Current Behavioral Status: Ricardo could be sarcastic at times. He could become easily agitated and disoriented. Thinking was often irrational. He enjoyed physical exercise and work of any kind. He enjoyed horses.

Funding and Discharge Options: Because he was injured in the line of duty, he was funded by Texas Workers Compensation. His current wife was unable to care for him at home with the additional responsibilities of the children, now both teenagers. Long-term care was a possibility to be considered.

DANICA: LIFE CLIENT TALLANGATTA COMPOSITE CLIENT

History Prior to the Injury: Danica was a 27-year-old white female. Her father was deceased, and her mother resided in a distant state at the time of this study. She was the eldest of four daughters. Danica was a high achiever until her junior year in high school. She had been elected "Class Favorite" during her sophomore year; however, shortly after that year she began experimenting with drugs. She had been an active volunteer reader for the blind prior to her drug habit which gradually caused her to deteriorate. She lacked direction in life and appeared disinterested in any activities.

Family History: All of Danica's family resided out of state; however, they stayed in touch and communicated regularly by mail. After the accident, she and her husband divorced. Her husband was rarely in contact with Danica or any of the family and provided no support at the time of this study, financially or emotionally.

169

Injury History: Six years ago, Danica and her husband were leaving on a routine weekend shopping trip when they were broadsided at an intersection. Danica was an unrestrained passenger in the front seat and was thrown through the windshield. She suffered multiple lacerations and fractures about the face. Her right femur was fractured as was her pelvis. She sustained an open brain injury to her right frontal lobe. She had left-sided upper and lower hemiparesis and walked with the aid of a cane.

Current Physical and Medical Condition: She had a shunt due to the hydrocephalus, secondary to the head injury.

Current Cognitive Status: Problem-solving skills were weak for this composite client. Danica had difficulty in initiation, judgment, and flexibility. Short-term memory needed to be strengthened.

Current Behavioral Status: With the exception of her inability to express her emotions and her propensity to sarcasm, Danica was stable behaviorally.

Funding and Discharge Options: Danica's funding was available through a trust fund established by her late father. Long-term care and a good quality of life were the treatment goals.

POSITIVE STAFF MEMBER COMPOSITE: COLTON CRISWELL

Colton was a tall, lanky, and handsome young Afro-American. He was probably 26- or 27-years-old having been out of college for the past five years. Colton received his degree in physical education from the university located in the small town not far from Epworth. He served as an intern at the rehabilitation network during his final year of school working with the Epworth clients on their physical education programs. He enjoyed the work and the personal satisfaction of helping the clients and excitedly accepted a full-time position following graduation. Colton was the youngest of three children; both older sisters were married with children of their own. Since he was a bachelor with no children, Colton doted on his nieces and nephews. Though his family lived within the surrounding university community, Colton resided in his own duplex and had an active lifestyle. This composite staff member was active in his church, refereed the YMCA youth sports, and enjoyed a full social calendar. During employment over the last five years, he had been promoted to a supervisory capacity earning the title of senior counselor. He continued to be active in the training programs offered, including the Brain Injury Specialist Certification and, at the time of this study, had begun his quest for his Master's degree in Physical Therapy.

Colton was a joy to work with as a staffer, and as a researcher I learned a great deal from him. His vivacious enthusiasm and sensitivity always seemed to generate an energy that defied explanation because he rarely moved other than in slow motion. Perhaps, it was the "unhurried," "not hassled," "all will be well, no matter what," calm that infused a room and gave the clients a sense of security. I noticed that when I had a question or concern, Colton was the one I sought for advice. I trusted him, and it was obvious the clients did as well for they too sought him in preference to other staffers. His interactions were never hurried with the clients; he always gave complete answers. Not to be fooled by his gentle nature, Colton stood his ground when necessary, 'the iron fist in a velvet glove.' A client never had to wonder where he or she stood in relation to Colton or his opinion of a behavior or decision. Often I stood across the room and just watched Colton work. He reminded me of a proud eagle guarding his nest. Under his watch, all clients and staff carried out their duties, being allowed to solve problems for themselves. However, if 'danger' looked imminent, for example a client was having difficulty balancing his checkbook, before it could reach crisis situation and become a demotivator to the client, Colton would swoop down from his watch and patiently explain each and every step along the way until the client was again confident to attempt the task alone. On several occasions, I paid particular attention to the content of Colton's conversations—then I knew the secret to his popularity: during the shifts I particularly monitored, over 85% of his interactions/comments were of a positive, complimentary, or socially engaging nature. He, indeed, made the clients feel like his friends. He treated them with the same respect he treated the staff, as equal human beings.

NEGATIVE STAFF MEMBER COMPOSITE: ANNA RATCHETT

Assistant Manager Anna Ratchett, what a character! I do believe deep down in her heart of hearts she was genuinely concerned for the clients and eager to help—it just did not always come across that way. My guess was that Anna was in her late 20s or very early 30s. This composite staffer, like Colton, also graduated from the local university. Her degree was in psychology. Anna was married with no children at the time of this study. She and her husband lived in a small community not far from the rehabilitation headquarters. The impression she left on me after our first meeting was that of a stereotypical "high school cheerleader." None of us, it seemed, were quite as good as she was in working with the clients. I did not know much about Anna's family or her outside activities as she was a very private, work competitive person. Anna, I believe, was very controlling. She wanted everyone, clients and staff alike, to report only to her. No activity or conversation escaped her. I always felt like a prison guard being watched closely by the warden when she was in charge. In other words, her ideas, suggestions, concerns, were more important than others', and she did not hesitate to tell us so in front of the clients. If the word flexible defined Colton, the word inflexible defined Anna. Anna seemed to be overbearing with the clients. She suffocated their enthusiasm by over-directing and not allowing them the normal pleasures that as humans we all enjoy, such as walking on a summer night, being a "couch potato" occasionally, or participating in a spur-of-the-moment activity. For example, a client was not allowed to enjoy a conversation with another client, or even staff without Anna inquiring about the nature of the conversation. I do not remember seeing her really laugh in the entire time I was on site. Several clients described her actions in the same way—"stifling."

Perhaps her actions conjured memories of my own days of feeling suppressed in rehabilitation situations, but I was always relieved to be able to work in an area other than under her supervision. Fellow staffers when frustrated told me "the room always seems tense when she walks in." Anna was very thorough in her organizational skills, something to be commended, but they just never seemed to leave room for "life."

The Model

"The purpose of grounded theory method is, of course, to build theory that is faithful to and illuminates the area under study" (Strauss and Corbin, 1990, p. 24). The grounded theory model, on a diagram, is a visual representation of the relationships among the concepts that create the theory. The model presented in Figure 5.1 represents my interpretation of the relationships present in this study as they evolved from Preliminary Studies 1 and 2. Since the inception of Preliminary Study 1, my knowledge of the synergistic nature of the phenomenon being investigated, motivation, has grown more sophisticated and ideas confirmed through multiple data sources. Therefore, unlike the static and unidimensional Preliminary Study models represented in Figures 3.1 and 3.2, the model for this study required a dynamic and multidimensional presentation. In this study of individuals with TBI, the outcome of motivation was *engagement* in rehabilitation programs. The data in this study suggested that engagement was achieved as a result of a synergy that was interactionally created by four contextual categories:

one's *perception of self, perception of recovery, vision,* and *personal interactions.* This synergy was called *momentum*, the central phenomenon. The interactional relationships of this study are represented in Figure 5.2. The outcomes of momentum generated continued rehabilitation, which, in turn, enabled the client to return to community life at the highest level possible for him/herself. Because of the complex nature of the interdependent parts of this study's model, I first present an overview of the central phenomenon, *momentum*, its relationship to the

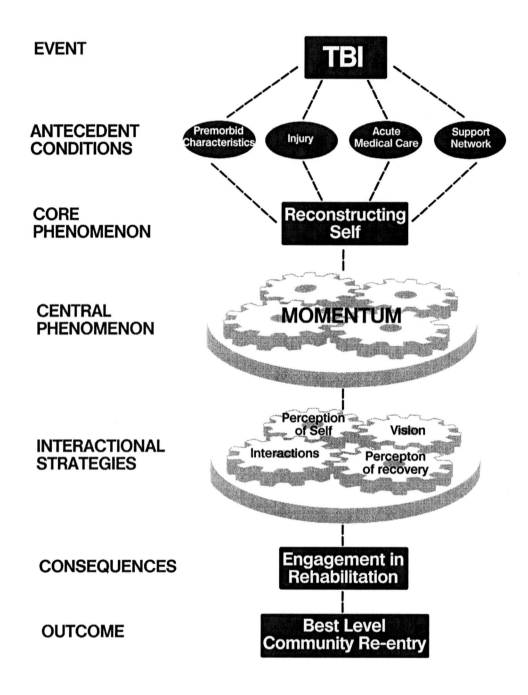

Figure 5.1.   Momentum: A grounded theory model

176

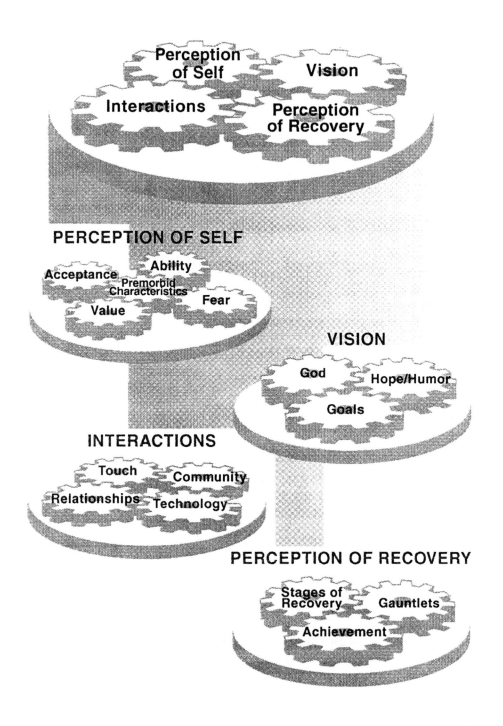

Figure 5.2. Interactional Strategies of Momentum

177

outcomes of the study, and its influence upon the architecture of the model. Next, I present an overview of the contextual categories. Following this diagrammatic introductory section, each of the contextual categories will be fully discussed. The conclusion of this chapter will feature case studies illustrating the model.

The Central Phenomenon

As noted by Prigatano and Schacter (1991), motivation has perhaps not been researched in depth due to the difficulty of time commitment as well as the rigors of making it fit into the controlled molds of conventional medical research. However, most researchers agree motivation is a key in the rehabilitation process for the individual with a traumatic brain injury (TBI).

"Health research is beginning a new phase [qualitative methodology], with questions that have never been addressed well, if at all, by conventional inquiry" according to Lincoln (1992, p. 390). This study used the "new phase" to study motivation.

The central phenomenon of a qualitative study is "the central idea, event, happening, incident about which a set of actions or interactions are directed at managing, handling, or to which the set of actions is related" (Strauss & Corbin, 1990, p. 96). The central phenomenon filters to the forefront as the data are analyzed. Arguably the direction of interest in any study is influenced by the theoretical orientations of the investigator and that does, to some extent, direct the outcome. However, it is critical that all outcomes be grounded in the data gathered. It is not uncommon for the emerging phenomenon from a set of data to

178

be different from the researcher's expectations, as was the case in this study. I entered into this study armed with a multitude of motivational theories from Descartes to Deci. I was poised to discover which of the three common divisions of motivation: biological, behavioral, or cognitive (Petri, 1991), held the secret for the individual with TBI. I was taken by surprise, then, to name none of these theories or areas as the central phenomenon, but rather the interaction of many facets. By interaction, I am meaning the "momentum" generated by events in one's life that sustains personal interest toward the action we see. By definition, momentum is "strength or force gained by motion or through the development of events" (Merriam-Webster, 1993, p. 750). Therefore, I have chosen to label the central phenomenon of this study *momentum*, which is divided into four major categories as they relate to the individual with TBI: self-perception, perception of recovery, vision, and interactions.

The momentum that is generated from the interaction of the above named categories propels the individual into personal commitment of action [volition] and effort in his/her rehabilitation. Therefore, the outcome, *engagement*, is the aggregate result of the interaction of the various named categories.

Victor Frankl (1984), speaking on success, noted: "For success, like happiness, cannot be pursued; it must ensue, and it only does so as the unintended side-effect of one's personal dedication to a cause greater than oneself or as the by-product of one's surrender to a person other than oneself." As the central phenomenon emerged, I could understand and apply the wisdom of Frankl for all the desires of rehabilitation workers longing for the successes of their clients: we can only teach, or encourage, or aim at motivation in individuals with TBI, we cannot pursue it. Motivation must ensue, and it only does so as the unintended side-effect, the momentum, the synergy that just happens when effortful behavior of rehabilitation becomes automatic.

The model evolved as I contemplated various ways in which one can see momentum. Analogies simple to complex, from a tire rolling down a hill to a steam engine, all crossed my mind; however, it was the definition of momentum itself that led me to select a gyroscope as my metaphor. A gyroscope is "a wheel or disk mounted to spin rapidly about an axis and also free to rotate...the entire apparatus offers considerable opposition depending on the angular momentum to any torque that would change the direction of the axis of spin" (Merriam-Webster, 1993, p. 520). For the individual recovering from TBI, momentum gained, if strong enough, can oppose the negative forces such as discouragement, disability, or depression to name a few. The metaphor will be illustrated following the discussion of the contextual categories.

Summary of Study Relationships

The antecedent conditions (premorbid characteristics, manifestation of the injury, support, and medical care) remained constant through Preliminary Study 1, Preliminary Study 2, and the main study. Likewise the major central phenomenon, "reconstructing self," has remained identical throughout these studies. This is not a contradiction of the above-named central phenomenon for this study, momentum, but rather recognition that, in fact, there were two salient phenomena present in this third study. As discussed by Strauss and Corbin, "it is essential, however, to make a choice between them …choose one phenomenon, relate the other category to it as a subsidiary category, then write it as a single theory" (1990, p. 121-122). Recall the grounded models of the preliminary studies, Figures 3.1, 3.2, and note that the motivational elements studied in this project were on the fringes of the previous studies and just did not emerge in any clearly definable nature. Finally, the contextual categories of "stages of recovery" in Preliminary Study 2 have now been refined as a portion of the individual's perception of recovery.

Preview of Outcomes and Contextual Categories

According to Strauss and Corbin, open coding fractures the data and allows one to identify some categories while axial coding puts those data back together making connections between a category and its subcategories (1990, p. 96-97). Following the statement of outcomes and the four primary contextual categories this section presents each category in detail in light of its subcategories and their properties.

OUTCOMES

The answer to the riddle "how does motivation occur?" has been elusive for centuries. While researchers have not been able to agree on the "how" of motivation, they have agreed on the "what," the outcome. The by-product of the motivated person has been labeled many things such as volition, determination, will, and conation. For this study, the outcome is labeled *engagement* in rehabilitation programs.

Engagement for an individual in rehabilitation exists along a continuum ranging from engagement (involvement, participation in rehabilitative activities) to disengagement (withdrawal from rehabilitative activities). Sustained positive emotions and behavioral activity during retraining are manifestations of an individual engaged in rehabilitation. The converse of such engagement (passivity, quickness to abandon an activity, and negative emotional and behavioral outbursts) is a picture of a disengaged individual. There appear to be six distinct stages along the engagement continuum: moving from most disengaged to most engaged—withdrawn, ritualistic, rebellious, conformist, innovative, and enmeshed (Connell, 1990, Connel & Wellborn, 1991). For this study, the outcome category of engagement seems to exhibit all the above qualities, yet offered another interesting characteristic of the engaged individual: reflectiveness.

The individual who achieves engagement has the ability to step back periodically and evaluate, reflect, upon his/her engagement. This evaluative or reflective characteristic allows the individual to learn from his/her previous experiences whether these experiences had a positive or negative outcome.

The consequence, then, is the maximum level of recovery possible for reentry into community-life for the individual with TBI. Just as no two brain injuries are identical, neither will any two community reentry levels be identical. However, if the momentum is sustained over a long enough period of time generating extended participation in rehabilitation efforts, then, the best possible outcome is more attainable for each individual.

SELF-PERCEPTION

Each of us lives with a set of personalized ideals for life, including our beliefs, our hopes, our fears, and our innermost thoughts. How we function day-to-day is dependent upon how we perceive ourselves personally and in relation to those around us. The individual with TBI is no different. Nochi (1997) examined the self-perception of individuals with TBI. His findings suggest that this population experiences a loss of self in various forms: loss of single self-history, the opaque self, the devalued self, and the labeled self. The dynamics of each of these areas are ones we face daily without thought given to our calculations for value; however, for the TBI individual, that automatic calculation is not so easy. The subcategories suggested in this research study for the value of self-perception are: ability, value, perception of premorbid self, acceptance of self as "injured," and fear.

PERCEPTION OF RECOVERY

As suggested in Study 2, the individual with TBI journeys through three stages in the recovery process. How an individual see him/herself in these stages has a great influence upon his/her ultimate outcome. The stages of recovery as defined in the earlier study were just one of the subcategories of 'perception of recovery' with properties of learning styles and assessment. The other subcategories of the recovery contextual category are: achievement and gauntlets, which are motivators and demotivators.

VISION

"Where there is no vision the people perish." (Proverbs 29:18a) The contextual category of vision is divided into three subcategories: spiritual vision, achievement visions (goals), and visions of hope/humor. It was interesting to observe the difference in those individuals with TBI who relied upon spiritual foundations and those who did not. While those who were connected to some spiritual belief in God still had plenty of frustrations and problems, there seemed to be a calm about them, even in crisis, that those without such recognition in life did not have. The presence of the spirit-filled life seemed to give a 'value' to the individual that sustained him/her in daily activities.

The common element in motivational studies since the beginning of such studies has been the link to the 'visions,' the goals of the individual for the future. This study was no different in that the value of goals was recognized as a subcategory within this contextual category. Vision was, however, no more or less important than the other three contextual categories. Only the individual can define the ideal for a "good quality of life" which in turn defines his/her goals. As discussed in Chapter 2, previous studies in the field of TBI recovery experienced research design problems, for goals that were good for one TBI individual were not necessarily good for another.

The final vision these data suggested was that of hope and humor. An individual's ability to cherish recovery with anticipation and the confidence of reaching a goal seemed critical to vision. Even the phenomenon of 'hope against hope,' that is, hope without any basis for expecting fulfillment of the hope, appeared valuable. Coupled with hope was the vision of humor. The age-old adage, 'laughter is the best medicine,' was obvious. Laughter seemed to fuel the energy of hope.

INTERACTIONS

We do not exist in a vacuum; therefore, our interactions with others and with resources in our environment are critical to our ultimate happiness and success in life. This fact is also true for the TBI population. The subcategories of this contextual category include: relationships, technology, touch, and community.

Discussion of Contextual Categories

SELF-PERCEPTION

From infancy we each construct a personal image of ourselves. We are molded by our environments. As we develop a picture of self that we like, we protect it, we remember it, we embrace it. The remembered self over the years can refer to our recollections of past concepts of self. Memory is a great contributor to self-actualization for it provides the raw data with which we build our images. However, our construction of self is not tethered to memory alone; new experiences can also alter our self-perceptions (Hirst, in Neisser & Fivush, 1994).

> New experience may alter self by buttressing existing themes, but often one cannot easily weave a present experience into the ongoing narrative without disturbing a narrative theme. A new experience might evoke new attitudes and beliefs...and may lead to an entire restructuring of the narrative" (pp. 253-254).

Hirst, in investigating the narrative self in amnesiacs, discovered that memory is not the only builder of our self-perceptions, but rather includes externalized and collective representations as well. This complex constructing of self is automatic, though perplexing at times, to each individual. However, the automaticity of this construction becomes labored following TBI and creates one of the greatest hurdles to the individual in rehabilitation. According to psychologists (Neisser, Baddeley, Hirst, Reed, in Neisser & Fivush, 1994), we each exhibit a self-representation (our story based upon explicit memories) and a self-presentation (our actions). For individuals with TBI, the conflict often exists between who they remember (or think they remember) they were premorbidly and the actions they now battle to control or perform. How one perceives him/herself impacts his/her ability to function in everyday life. The inertia, the force of being in control of oneself, is a key to generating a positive perception of self. This study suggested that there are five subcategories (each capable of affecting this personal inertia) to the element of perception of self: premorbid representation, ability, value, acceptance of injury, and fear, as illustrated in Figure 5.3.

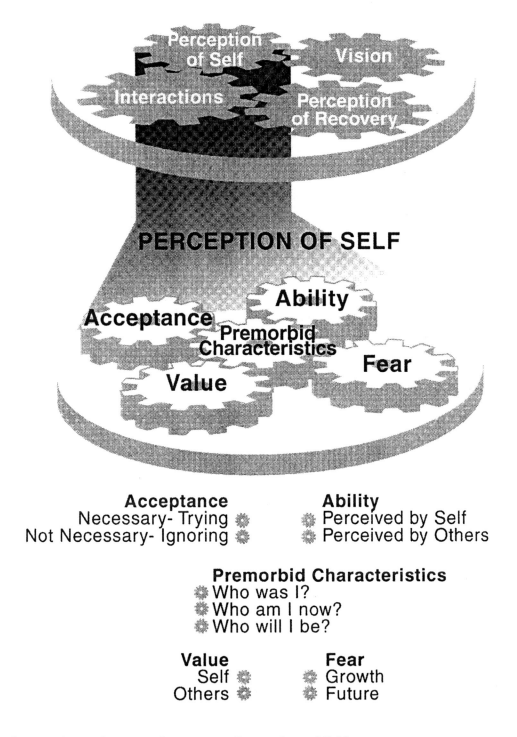

Figure 5.3.   Contextual category: Perception of Self

Premorbid Representation

As illustrated in Figure 5.3, the emergent subcategory of premorbid representation rests in the center of the model, representing its central impact upon the self-perception of individuals with TBI. There seems to be no disagreement whatsoever among researchers in any field that the premorbid characteristics of an individual greatly affect his/her life after TBI. Characteristics from simple demographics (such as age, gender, or race) to the more complex indicators (such as IQ, social environment, or personal values) each mold the resurgence of the individual in rehabilitation. These accepted premises, however, are not the properties of this subcategory, rather the properties for consideration were TBI individuals' answers to three questions: (1) Who was I? (2) Who am I now?, and (3) Will I be the same, worse, or better than I was? While the individual with TBI grapples with these questions in a cyclical fashion, the cycle generally follows the order named. The individual's inner response to his/her premorbid self affects his/her post-injury growth. "Well, I never really accepted it…. Even now,…I protect my ego" claimed Stan who was frustrated because he was not the same person and may not or cannot return to the former self. He clung to his former self and held expectations for himself that hindered his rehabilitation process, for he would not recognize the validity of related activities such as exercise. The opposite response could be seen in Joe, who was elated because he felt he was a better person because of his injury and subsequent rebirth, and this feeling was reflected in his general cooperative nature in rehabilitation activities:

Joe: "I might say, I think that it's really a stressful question. I'll answer the best I can. I feel better now than I was when I was better at home."

L: "Do you really? That's good. I like that answer."

Joe: "See, if I was home not having a head injury, I would probably be very upset. If there's nothing wrong with me. Everything's fine. That kind of like pulls on you. It just doesn't matter—I'd rather stay the way I am now."

L: "So, you're happier now in yourself?"

Joe: "Yes."

L: "Why?"

Joe: "Cause I don't love my Dad…I was not happy before my accident. I was always mad at myself. I never want to be the person I was in the past because I don't like that feeling in myself. I feel there's nothing wrong with me [now] and just go on."

Ruth, a long-term client offered some insight into the struggle of an individual in considering her premorbid self: "Your life is going in one direction and all of a sudden you are going in the opposite direction. You had no control over the change—you had no control over the change. None—it just happened. … After a period you realize you're not getting anywhere. No miracles. You have to do it. Wake-up—the same each day, you finally realize it's you that has to do something."

Perhaps the clearest picture of the on-going struggle year after year that an individual with TBI faces was offered by Ray and Hugh, clients at the Tallangatta program:

Ray: And so, that's [attempting college again] what I was doing when [personal contact] had come and kind of talked to me and said "well, we have a thing in [state] set up called Epworth. And it's a new thing. It's sort of like a preliminary program. And we would like very much for you,

189

since you have a traumatic brain injury to come there and see what happens." And I've been here for 11 years—11 years! And the thing is, I don't like to admit this but I am without a clue. I am successful at this but I would like to be in a situation where I'm completely free every day to do other things. And possibly be successful at them. Rather than just, you know, it's very good. You know, they've seen one thing that works, that is a working thing, like the structure. And you know what's going to happen all the time. That works but 10 years! 10 years! 12 years! I've been doing that. And it works. I'm completely content and happy because it works. And then, what I was doing didn't work 12 years. And what I am doing now works but—you know, I don't know…

L: So, you're saying that you'd like to try something different besides just…

Ray: Yes, but I'd like to remain successful. Because I found from the time I was born 'til now I enjoy the feeling of being successful. And one thing that I spent 20 years at and was very successful at, suddenly I wasn't successful at it any more. So, now, I've spent another, like 15 years, from something I was successful at and but I'm saying, it's like…(long pause)

L: …going in a different direction.

Ray: Yeah. Like an arc. Say you have an arc and you're figuring the degrees of the arc by measuring the amount of each angle and you find out how the arc works. But that doesn't work any more, so you're saying, 'okay, I'll do something else.' And you figure out how this arc works, too. But, those arcs will never intersect. So, I was always trying, I've been trying to intersect the arcs that will not intersect.

L: Okay!

Ray: The difficulty—the right hand—it needs to be dealt with rather than just saying, 'you should act like' the doctor blah, blah, blah. There's a perfect example of what I'm talking about. I was in the hospital and in a day room and I said to the doctor, cause the doctor would come in and talk to me, and I said, 'well I used to play a guitar. I have 3 really nice guitars. And I used to play in a band. And now, I can't do that. I can't—my ability to comprehend the situation is not—it's like a radio tuner that's off the station. And you're trying to do it and you can't get it.' And so, he said, "let me put it in perspective for you. You should be very, very happy that you know what a guitar is." So, now, one person says this, that I should be happy I know what a guitar is. I'm saying, I can't play the music I used to play on my guitar. So,

Hugh: That's happened to me. I used to play guitar before my accident and I can't now. I just forgot how. And so, I just kind of gave it up and I kept saying I would do it and I don't. You know, it's not a big deal to me now. It's just trying to get better. Now, something else. The first five jobs I had, I was a cook, all right, in different restaurants. My last job I had, I worked for an insurance company, all right? Now, I had my accident and I can't go back to work with that insurance company right now. It's kind of like your first job, you know. And, so, I'm back to start working at fast-food restaurants like I am now. It's like two magnets— you know you can't put them together. You know, cause they repel, just like his arcs, he talking about, they won't go together. It's frustrating...

Both of these young men were struggling to figure out just what skills they had regained and what direction they could expect from life. Both longed to be successful and neither knew exactly what skills were most marketable. They had become successful with the structure of the rehabilitation network and were growing restless for a new challenge. Their assessment of progress was their way of gauging individual potential.

Ability

Listening to the above conversation, one can quickly surmise that the individuals with TBI were frustrated attempting to match their past experiences and their current abilities. The brain-injury population in this study had cognitive reasoning abilities at some level, and individuals attempted to evaluate their abilities as the normal population does, against society. One of the residential individuals at Windy Hill, a mid-level program, offered this assessment of his ability:

EC: Oh yes! I've experienced the—depressed and the helplessness. But I've also turned right back around—I have switched. By gosh, he can do it, I can do it.

L: Okay.

EC: And I myself, I am especially—came into this way of thinking because of my age. In other words, Glenn here, hey, say for instance, hey, okay, he can run a 5K or a 10K in 20 minutes. Well, by gosh, if that young whippersnapper can, by gosh, I can.

L: But you're older than that young whippersnapper.

EC: I know. That means I'm more experienced.

L: Oh, okay. So, to you, more experience makes it better.

EC: Well, somewhat.

L: Okay.

EC: However, I mean, it does, well, experience is good. However, let's face reality. Okay. He has a whole lot better because of his age—he should be able to go longer than myself.

L: Okay.

EC: Because, well, I'm twice his age. Okay. So, therefore, he ought to be able to go at least a third longer, really....(snip)

The inner drive to prove we have the ability to accomplish a task is a strong motivator for any individual. Another lifelong client, though severely injured, reflects his desire for his abilities and physical improvement to be recognized. In a split second his life and family were snatched from him and now, over 20 years later, he is still seeking the recognition of his desire and ability to provide for his family:

(conversation took place while walking the track—transcription begins deep into a detailed description of injuries)

Jeff: And from right here to right here, I got a plate in my head.

L: You're incredible! So, do you see from week to week, do you feel like you're getting better? Or do you still feel like after all these years, you're—oh, for lack of a better word, let's use the word, recovering....

Jeff: Yeah, well, I consider myself sometimes, but my eyesight, I think's getting a little better, some days. Some days, I don't know. I don't know....

L: Do you find that things like your memory get any better?

Jeff: Yeah, it gets better. I kinda consider myself here I'm at, where I stay at, you know. And, well I'm considering on getting me a job somewhere, but I kinda back off of it, and all that, my wife don't know, I like to tell her what I'm thinking about. But every time I want to talk to her, I back off from it.

L: What you're thinking about...you mean getting a job?

Jeff: Yeah.

(snip conversations with other TBI walkers)

Jeff: ...I just want to try to get him [Dr. Rutledge] to see if he would—if I could go back from—just like leaving Windy Hill and go to the Woodshop home and from home to Woodshop. See if I could, you know, do it that way.

L: So, in other words, let you live at home with your wife?

Jeff: Yeah, go back and forth to work that way. I know that's a big deal to say, but...

L: I think that's a great goal. I don't have any problem with that. That's a super goal. What does your wife say about that?

Jeff: I haven't told her yet.

L: I think I'd tell her first. That's the courteous thing to do. Plus if you've discussed it with her, see, then it's kind of more of a family type thing. But, certainly a married man would want to be with his wife.

Jeff: Yeah, I wanna—I don't know what's really come over me. I'm different.

L: How?

Jeff: Uh, I noticed that I …I… I can't help myself every time I'm around my wife. I want to make sure she's got enough stuff. I was thinking—now, it's silly of me to think this—but it ain't though—I was thinking about giving her money where she can get her clothes for her, adornments and stuff. Put it that way.

L: Why would that be silly?

Jeff: I don't think it is…I know it. And all the money I get from the Woodshop, I want to give to her.

Clearly, Jeff is longing to fulfill his manly responsibilities to his wife, to be the provider, the caregiver, the friend, the lover. Individuals with TBI, like Jeff, are continually assessing their ability and progress in light of society standards. This inner drive to remain competitive in life is a key ingredient of generating momentum.

Value

It appears that in defining our perception of self our abilities and our value are inextricably bound. From exasperation to exultation our feelings for our value and how we are valued affect our self-perception.

As Joe and I were chatting one day, he commented, "People just don't understand. People just don't see that—the real you. It doesn't matter. People doesn't matter any more. It just don't work. People like discard you, throw you

194

away, give you a lot of trouble." More than once, Ellis declared to me, "...you're one of us, so you know I'm worth something, a lot of these guys like [staff names] treat me like I'm worth nothing. They can't really understand. You can, you've been there. Do you ever hurt inside 'cuz you're not understood on the outside?" The individual with TBI often begins early in recovery affirming his/her value as did Windy, approximately one year post-injury, during her initial interview: "I'm just like everyone else, forget I've had a brain injury." Paula offered insight to value in one simple sentence: "Give me credit for what I am—what I was. What I was in the past."

The agony of feeling without value to others faded as the individual with TBI gained some levels of achievement in his/her new life, as illustrated in this conversation of Terri and one of the members of the Epworth review team on Rutledge Day.

> Terri: Yeah. I wait more tables than I am—oh my goodness, I'm running and moving and—my manager told me to go back to her desk and sit down for 5 minutes and take a breather. And I did. I didn't say, 'oh, no, no, I can handle it.' I just did as I was told. And because everyone was calling my name—the phone was going off the hook. We had people coming in, we had people waiting to be seated, we didn't have any tables available. We had people, you know—it was just nuts. It was mad.

> Inez: Now, when people eat the buffet, do you get tips because you bring their drinks and stuff like that?

> Terri: Yes.

> Valerie: Yes, well they're supposed to tip. Not everyone understands the tipping process...(all laugh) Bet you understand it a lot more now! Right?

> Terri: Oh, yes I do! And so, it's not a matter of—it's not free money. It definitely is not free money because we're making sure that—I mean,

we wait. I mean, we're making sure that your drinks are full and that you have extra napkins and that we're trying to kind of read your mind before you have a need or a want. So, it's interesting. And then, even on the buffet, we're saying, 'Is there anything we can get you? Is there anything that you might want?' You know, 'How is everything?' It's that kind of thing. It's real interesting. It's scary. It's scary at times.

Inez: Sure! You know I think what is most amazing is how well you handled a change in your structure. ...

Terri: Thank you!

(snip)

Terri: I have some more good information.

Inez: What's that?

Terri: While I was at work I got a call from the Grill and said that they wanted me to come in. I mean, they—and I was like, 'What?' I said, 'no, thank you, I've already received another job.' And they said, 'Well, do you have any friends that are like you because we would like somebody with your qualities?' and it just, you know, I felt really good about that.

Acceptance of being "injured"

As Terri battled for her perception of personal value and ability, she was also struggling with the fact that she was injured. The struggle individuals experience in attempts to accept their injury can be seen in the manner in which they reflect upon events in this following conversation. Note the suggestions for assisting other individuals with TBI past personal struggles. During this reflection, also note the introspective nature of the conversation as highlighted by italics. Those struggles are fraught with emotion as noted in the bolded text.

Paula: Give them [individuals with TBI] credit and talk to them. Get to know them. It's all like Dr. Rutledge says, it takes time. Become friends with them. Cause God I hated it so bad. Here I still do sometimes

196

whenever some staff or doctor or nurse would tell me what to do and expect me to bow my head and say, 'yes, ma'am.' You know, treat them like they're people. And remember they have feelings, too. Treat them like they're human.

L: Good point. So, you're nodding your head. What would you say, Terri?

Terri: I agree with that. I would say give them time. That there's a waiting period for them to accept the information that's given. I know I've gone through a lot myself of not quite understanding. Even though I was told I was brain injured, you know, three years ago. *I was like, didn't believe them. Because I would look in the mirror and I saw this girl and I wasn't disfigured and I saw…*

Paula: You looked the same.

Terri: *… I looked, well, I had shorter hair. But, I mean, I pretty much looked the same. I wasn't scarred up. And I didn't understand about—* okay, for instance, I didn't understand how my brain controlled my entire body and since being here and since learning about how the brain controls the functions of my entire body, I feel so much more knowledgeable about the processes. And about—since I've had seizures, I've really appreciate—have come to appreciate the staff in realizing that they're not the enemy any more. That they are here to help and that they are here to supervise me in a way that won't lead me into dangerous situations. **Whereas before I was like just putting up with it—just doing okay. 'Okay, whatever you say.' And I was thinking to myself, 'Now, get the hell out of my face.'** But I wasn't agreeing with what they were saying or doing. I was just trying for the moment, 'okay, whatever.' And then, but that wasn't helping. And so, there's a time and for every person, this time period is different. It took me, oh my goodness, pretty much 30 years—30 years to finally—when I had a grand mal, …

Acceptance was a process for most individuals with TBI. Knowing

growth was a major contributor in acceptance, it was easy to distinguish the

"young" brain-injured individuals in this conversation from the "seasoned" ones.

The following conversation, though lengthy, illustrates the growth of each TBI survivor and the strength of a solid rehabilitation environment with strong leadership and camaraderie among clients.

In the initial portion of the conversation, note the brevity of Myrtle's answer. Myrtle has not been injured long and is just beginning to seek answers. Toward the end of this first section of conversation, Myrtle offers the expected responses for indication of acceptance; however, in the second section of the conversation, note her questioning of another on how to achieve acceptance. Todd and Richard are seasoned survivors, each 11 years' post-injury. Richard is six years older than Todd. Note the depth of Richard's answer in this first section:

> L: Now, I have had people tell me that one of the most important things about getting over a head injury is that you've got to accept the disability before you can make any progress.
>
> Myrtle: That is true.
>
> Todd: That is very true. You've got to accept that you're hurt—you were hurt and that you have a certain physical problem or weight problem, eating habits are poor….
>
> L: Okay. What do you think happens if you don't accept it?
>
> Todd: It just makes it longer and harder for you to…
>
> Richard: You find out the hard way.
>
> L: You find out the hard way?
>
> Richard: Delay things later and keep going, going and they going to go very, very fast and deal with the problem. Like driving full speed ahead and going into brick walls.
>
> L: So, you think if they don't accept it, they try to go full speed ahead. Is that what you're saying, Richard?
>
> Richard: Yes, that is, if they don't accept it.

L: Do you remember a time, after your own accident, that you perhaps did not accept the fact that you had a problem? Can you remember when you started accepting it?

Richard: I can believe I was a little on the hard-headed side...

L: You, hard-headed, Richard?

Richard: A little while back, but not usually anywhere as much now at least.

L: Okay. Good. So, why are you not as hard-headed now?

Richard: Cause I have seen there are many friendly people around here. And who are willing to help us with whatever we need assistance with.

L: Okay. Good. Okay. Myrtle: what about you? Do you think you need to accept it? You're pretty new at the head injury game.

Myrtle: Yes, I am extremely new. I didn't think that I needed to accept my disability, but maybe I do a little more than I have been.

L: Okay. Do you think that you've accepted any part of your disability so far?

Myrtle: I've really learned to accept it. I know not all of it because I know I haven't accepted it all to the extent that I could but I believe that I've accepted pretty well.

L: Pretty well, part of it. What part would you say you've accepted?

Myrtle: Just not being able to do as much.

Myrtle is giving the expected response about acceptance, but her behavior and words did not quite match at the time of this study. However, note her comment to Bill, a survivor of many years and a resident in the supported community living program, Epworth's highest client level. She is seeking. Bill, on the other hand, has resolved the issue in his head and is now onto other matters.

He is a man of a few words in speaking of the past. He seems to have accepted the deficits and forged ahead, the ultimate goal for acceptance in recovery.

> L: Okay. Not being able to do as much. Bill, you're out there pretty much back into the community. Can you remember when you did or did not accept it?

> Bill: Well, I—the staff used to tell me to do something. I'd turn around and I talk negative to them. I told them I didn't want to do it. I learned that, you know what? I turned around cause I needed help.

> L: So, you didn't really accept it until after you came to Epworth?

> Bill: yeah.

> Myrtle: So, will you please tell me how?

> L: How is it that you accepted it after you came to Epworth? What was it about Epworth that made you accept it?

> Bill: The help from the staff and staff giving me information and stuff like that.

Todd concludes this conversation, perhaps best captures the struggles every survivor faces, the battle of recognizing the problems one day, and not the next.

> L: Todd, what made you accept it? When did you accept it do you think?

> Todd: Well, I accepted it was when I woke up from the coma and I saw myself hooked up to all these machines and I asked my Mom and Daddy what happened. They go, "You got hurt." And I looked at my girlfriend and I shook my head. And I said, "no, that's not true. This morning I was just with Natalie and I've been with her all day. I just took a nap this afternoon." My Mom said, "No, you're—see in the morning right now and it's 2 1/2 months later." What month are we? We're in May, aren't we? No, we're in the middle of August. What?

> L: Wow!

Todd: When I looked at my girlfriend, my girlfriend goes, "Yes, Todd you were almost killed on the street." And she said the name. And I go, "What?" she goes, no, no, no, no, he was the one driving the car that hit you when you were going home.

L: So, you pretty well accepted it from the time you woke up out of your coma? Did you ever have any problem accepting that you had a problem.

Todd: Yeah. I just, I tried to show lots of people that, like everybody, that I didn't have a problem. There was nothing wrong with me. Even when I was in a wheelchair and I wasn't walking alone. I needed staff—someone holding on to me, make sure I didn't lose my balance too bad, well, then, I wouldn't accept a staff or my Mom or Dad holding on to me make sure I wouldn't fall when I walked. I had to walk alone.

L: So, you're saying there were periods that you did accept it. And then periods that you did not accept it. And you kind of fluctuated back and forth?

Todd: Yeah.

Just as the timing of acceptance varied, so did the belief that "acceptance" of the injury had to come before progress. While at least 12 of the individuals with whom I worked agreed that acceptance did not necessarily have to come first, in different conversations, Chip and Stan were most opinionated on this issue but for differing reasons. First, note the response of Chip indicates that acceptance is (or can be) actually a by-product of beginning successful recovery .

Chip: …I think that acceptance should be one of the later steps is because first the person's got to learn to do is—the hardest thing for people to do is to accept something—they tend to push that step off 'til later, 'til until they're a lot better. And say, oh, yeah, I was hurt a while back, but I'm fine now. But, I think that acceptance is a part but it shouldn't be the first stage. I think that first stage should be relearning basic skills are required and then from there—I mean, cause if you try telling somebody's that's just been hurt, that they've had a head injury. More than likely I'll get cursed and I may get punched up side the head because they're not cognitively restructured yet. And I think that biggest

201

thing to work on first is the cognitive restructuring and then, go to acceptance that yes, you did have a head injury.

Stan, on the other hand, refused to accept the injury as a way of protecting who he was.

L: Stan, how do you respond to that acceptance theory?

Stan: Well, I never really accepted it. Even now, actually in a way I'm laid back. It's good because I protect my ego. It's just not accepting it. I won't.

L: You protect your ego?

Stan: Yeah.

L: Okay. Not accepting it protects your ego of what? Who Stan was?

Stan: Yeah.

L: Stan, the college student?

Stan: Yeah and the actor.

L: Okay.

Stan: Yes. Appearance is very important.

L: Your looks are important, okay. …What would you ultimately like to do?

Stan: Be on my own.

L: Be on your own?

Stan: I will be on my own.

L: You will be on your own, okay. How can you be on your own, though, if you can't drive and you can't cook and…

Stan: I can cook but …

202

(snip)

L: So, you're telling me it's not important for you to accept that you've had some disability that you've been left with from your accident.

Stan: I—it's important cause you only get better when you accept it.

L: Okay, then why—if you're telling me now that if you're going to get better when you really accept it, when are you going to accept it?

Stan: Yeah. I'm not saying that I know that I'm never going to accept it.

L: Okay, how are you going to get better then?

Stan: Just from repetition.

L: Just from repetition?

Stan: Yeah.

Stan's philosophy reflects the self-protective devices often used by survivors of TBI, ignore it and it will go away. Over time, then, the deficits slowly sink in and one comes to accept the need for compensatory strategies in order to survive back in the community. The denial, or lack of acceptance, is often a self-preservation of personal value technique more than it is a real denial.

Fear

The fear of what unknown qualities were associated with being TBI survivor seemed to hamper acceptance and the fear of the unknown qualities of an independent life often slowed community reentry attempts in the later stages of rehabilitation. Easily over 70% of the individuals with whom I worked could get so excited in conversation about their goals of independent living again—until the dialogue narrowed to the logistics of their declaration of independence. At the mid-level facility, Windy Hill, these conversations usually became derailed with discussion of their color category ("I can't possibly think about it now, I'm not in the right color category.") or physical limitations ("I'm still using a cane, I can't be independent."). By the time the individual had progressed to the Tallangatta program where independent living could become a reality, the variety of fear was manifested in discussions of life without the network of the rehabilitation facility staff, loss of insurance dollars by making too much money, lack of self-confidence, and simply that lump of fear that grips any of us when we leave home. The inner struggle seen in a conversation amongst Ray, Cecilia, and Hugh perhaps offered the best picture of the gripping fear of recovery and a move toward independence. Fear comes in different disguises for the survivor.

L: What will motivate you to move on?

Cecilia: Well, a guy that I—Someone who is intelligent like in that movie, Good Will Hunting. It's like Will—that's what I mean, someone who lives up to my dream. My hope person…

L: Okay. So, in other words, a relationship would be important to you.

Cecilia: Yeah.

L: Okay. That's fair.

Cecilia: It doesn't have to be that but, like,—for me to, like, be stable— for me to see myself able to do whatever to be a teacher, or whatever. I've got to have that somebody to come home to who wants me.

L: Okay. That's fair enough. So, how about you?

Hugh: I mean, I am doing better than I was since I've been here. And I'm my own guardian. And I could leave—I'm doing a lot of procrastinating now and you know. I'm just kind of like hanging out here and people say, 'if you're your own guardian, why don't you just leave?' I say, 'cause I have nowhere to go.' All right. I have nowhere to go and I'm just staying here and doing what I'm doing all the time.

L: Do you want to leave?

Hugh: Sure, I do. I mean I talked to my folks about it maybe a month or two ago—just say two. And they didn't think that I would do well out there on my own. That staying here was better. Of course, I didn't like that but they both said it. But I talked to them on different phone calls.

L: Why did they think that you did not want to—that you wouldn't do well out there?

Hugh: I don't know why. Now, they both said, if I was out there on my own, I'd wind up going to jail. Right!

L: Okay. So, but you don't think you would.

Hugh: No.

L: Okay. And you do want to leave some time? So, you're saying you do want to leave some time.

Hugh: Sure I do.

L: So, what would it take to make you get there? What's going to motivate you to stop procrastinating to get out?

Hugh: (long pause and sigh) I just need to, I need to look for stuff like wanting to be out on my own. Have a place to go, a good job and all that. And, instead of waiting for it to come to me. If I stay here, if I want to move into an apartment, you know, I can wait until they tell me I can go over there, or I can tell myself that I want to talk to them about going over there.

L: Good point!

Hugh: And I'll get over there sooner.

L: Good point! So, it's taking control.

Hugh: Right. Like [staff] said the other day, she said, they were talking about apartments out loud and she said my name and she said, 'You know, Hugh wanted to go to an apartment, see?' And I just don't come to that and say that. I just, like I say, procrastinate. And I know I can do it, I just don't. That's my problem.

L: Now, you've hit on something that's the key thing in rehab period. That's "how do we get people to move from there to there?"

The above discussion moved similar to many held during this study, that is, the clients would discuss their fears, desires, thoughts on progressing in recovery, often analyzing their growth. Then, almost without exception, the conversation would turn to attempts to put the final piece of their rehabilitation puzzle in place, what actually had to happen for them to be promoted back to the real world? The pattern for this discussion is illustrative for most other conversations held, that is, the clients' perception of recovery has a great bearing upon their progress. If the client is pursuing an unobtainable goal, then, in time, he/she will become frustrated to the level of giving up.

L: Ray, what would motivate you? Do you ever want to be out of here? You were a med student at the time you were hurt. What's it going to take to get you to the next level of accomplishment?

(snip)

Ray: You are asking me something I really wish I had a really concrete answer for you, but I don't think anyone at this table does even though we'd all like to. You're absolutely correct. We're all saying, if you have the answer, why don't you please tell me.

Cecilia: Patience—that's a great answer.

L: Okay. He's been patient for 12 years. How many more years? Okay, I've been patient for 13 years.

Cecilia: Exactly! Like, yeah.

L: Okay. Let's back up and look at it from another way. How do you define recovery?

Cecilia: A change of mind for me. A change of mind set.

(snip)
Ray: …to be content to be able to look at the situation and be content with the situation. And say, okay, I'm fine with this. It's completely fine with me that this is where I am. I'm not saying, 'well, this is what I could be.' You know.

Ray finally captures the essence of the unspoken goals of many in rehabilitation situations, knowing your capacity for success and finding your new 'niche' in society. At some point in the rehabilitation of each individual, he/she grows weary of the process and is ready to test the waters of society again. Most of the time, the clients participating in these three studies acknowledged that they would be content, even grateful, with a supported community or even group home situation if they knew for sure they could not be independent. The opportunity to test the water is paramount to the recovering individual. As the discussion continued, Hugh rose from his chair and graphically defined recovery.

Note: The following section of this conversation revolved around the illustration in Figure 5.4. *Hugh drew the boxes as he spoke, indicated in the text. Box letter designations are mine, not his.*

207

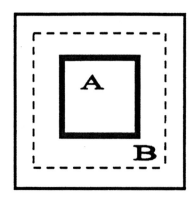

Figure 5.4. Hugh's Box

Hugh: I want to—well, it's kind of hard to get back where you were—but, I need to write this down. This is where I was before. (draws Box A) I want to get back there, you know. Not out here by it (draws Box B). It's hard to get back where you were and be with the friends you were with and same job—it's what I want to do but I can't but I want to get close (draws dotted line).

Ray: That's absolutely correct.

L: Okay. So, what Ray is saying, then, if we use this—if I'm understanding you right. Ray is saying, this is where I was and this is where I am now. I know I can never get back here but if I could learn to be happy right here—is that what you're saying?

Ray: That's what I'm saying. That's exactly what I'm saying. In fact, it is a definite learned thing that you don't long for something that is no longer around you. It is a learned thing to accept the reality that's right here and right now as, you know, cause that's all that there is. To understand that right here, right now is all that there is.

L: Okay. So, are you're telling me then, that you're not ultimately happy for the rest of your life. That you're in good health now, than….

Ray: That's what I would like to be. I would like to say, 'look! I'm able to walk. I don't need to have help breathing any more. I don't need to walk with a crutch. I don't have to wear hearing aids in both ears. And I don't need to have glasses on."

L: Okay. But are you telling me, then, that—when you were saying a while ago up here that you're looking for these arcs that don't intersect, are you telling me that—when you mention that you're tired of—that you like the structure to change a little bit, to know. Okay. You need it works right here. You're successful. Well, what about right here? Could you work and be successful? Are you saying that for the rest of your life, you're not content at this point to stay here working in Wood Shop?

Ray: But what I need to do is—what I'd like to do is be okay with that. Learn because since I don't know it, I don't think I'll ever know it. But getting to a point where I am accepting of my situation at this time. But see, that way keep me from progressing. People say the only way you can progress is to look for something in the future, you know,….

Hugh: …we need to understand how we're going to be happy at the dotted line.

In reality, the fears of individuals with TBI are no different facing life in

the community than any of ours. We are socially constructed individuals, and we

need that support structure around us. Darrell and Allan state:

Darrell: That's a big world out there. I like to have friends around. Here we've got friends. We've got moral support.

Allan: A family—it's like a family.

Darrell: …and when we leave, for moral support, you know we've got our folks at home to call on but we still have these people to call to when if we ever need it. But we still have that moral support. That's why I think it keeps us here—to find that moral support. It keeps everybody here and helping everybody in the program. Like I said, we help, every client helps every client.

Sometimes, the only thing we have to fear is fear itself. Even in

rehabilitation, when we can define the fear, we can begin to overcome it.

PERCEPTION OF RECOVERY

"Life by the yard is hard, by the inch it's a cinch." I could not begin to count the times during my life my mother recited that line to me; however, I can name the precise moment I saw it for its worth. It was a hot August day, 1997, and I was in the early days as a researcher on this project. I was touring Epworth and met a handsome young man named Neal. As I was chatting with this young man, 16 years post-injury, I saw emerging a picture of motivation from his perspective. Neal, in all probability, will forever be confined to his wheelchair—not from spinal damage, but rather from damage to the cortex of his brain that tells his legs to work. Neal suffered injury to the brain stem cerebellar complex with diffuse axial injury throughout the cortex. His speed of processing any outgoing information was painfully slow. However, in spite of all this, he was happy, hardworking in the rehabilitation program, and always asking for more time on the parallel bars, "I know with more time, I'll be able to walk." What drove him? What was his vision of recovery? Obviously, it was different from those of the rehabilitation workers assisting him. Neal will forever be special to my understanding of motivation for the TBI individual. He taught me with his quick wit, his winsome smile, and his simple philosophy the complex truth of recovery, that it had many parts.

Graphically illustrated in Figure 5.5, the contextual category of Perception of Recovery has three subcategories: stages of recovery, achievement, and gauntlets.

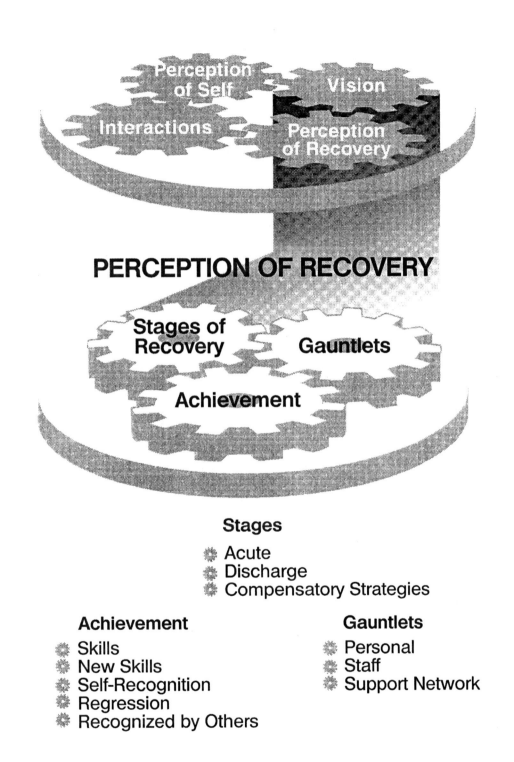

Stages
* Acute
* Discharge
* Compensatory Strategies

Achievement
* Skills
* New Skills
* Self-Recognition
* Regression
* Recognized by Others

Gauntlets
* Personal
* Staff
* Support Network

Figure 5.5. Contextual category: Perception of recovery

Stages of Recovery

As discussed in Chapter 3, Preliminary Study 2 presents three stages of recovery experienced by the individual with TBI. These participants seemed to agree that recovery cycled through three major stages:

1. Acute – point of injury to medical stabilization

2. Discharge (a new life) – may be simple like leaving the hospital for home or a rehabilitation center or complex like returning to work. The fact remains that once the individual has been discharged from the hospital and is medically stable, he/she is well and now must begin to mold a new life coping with the deficits remaining.

3. Compensatory Recovery – getting on with a new life.

The clients each had humorous anecdota of their movement through the stages whether it be from the initial acute stage or the triumphant compensatory recovery stage. One of the resident anecdotalists at Windy Hill recounts his realization of entry into Stage 2, discharge (a new life), as illustrated by the italics in this passage:

> EC: Uh. Actually when I felt helpless was in December whenever I went home {following his accident}—*I went home for Christmas. I was able to—I recovered enough that I could go home for Christmas.* And I went home for Christmas and I couldn't go out and look at my yard, my kids. *I could not, in other words, there was so many couldn'ts*—you can't do this, you can't do that—*what in the hell can I do?* Oh, you can do housework. You can pick up the dishes here. You can wash the dishes there. Well, excuse the way I'm wording this, but, that's not always been one of my preferences is to be a housewife. (laughs)

The individual with TBI seems to cycle through these stages based on the balance of three further subcategories: their personal perception of their recovery efforts at any given point, individual learning styles, and personal assessment of progress.

Personal Perception of Recovery

The stages of recovery suggested in Preliminary Study 2 were supported in this study in an unexpected manner. I worked with 30 Windy Hill clients for an extensive amount of time in my observation/work week. These clients were still working on adjustment to TBI, even though many were years removed from the injury itself. The Windy Hill clients had a mixture of behavioral, physical, and cognitive deficits. Each client responded to the question, "How will you know you are recovered" with the same type response, for example, "I'll be able to use my hand," "I'll not have to use this cane," "I'll be able to control my temper," "My shoulder will work," "I won't have the tremors." Each response was of a physical nature, although Stan did quip, "I could like name all the states in reverse alphabetical order" as a parting shot. The description given by the participants in Preliminary Study 2 for the characteristics of Stage 2 recovery were just that, physical in nature. Preliminary Study 2 participants felt they never were aware of the need to rectify cognitive deficits until Stage 3. The 25 clients at the Tallangatta program with whom I spent a great deal of time, each named a cognitive function such as "memory," "organizational skills," or "problem-solving skills," as their "recovery indicator." While these clients mentioned the improvement of some physical weakness or deficit, such as gait, or speech as a secondary indicator, none indicated a physical characteristic as their primary

213

indicator. One interesting fact of the movement of an individual between Stages 2 and 3 was the uncertainty with which one leapt to the next stage to the comfort zone of knowing you could return to Stage 2 and try again:

Richard: It's going to take a lot of time. And when I say it's going to take time ..like around years, I say, my God, next week. The hell with it. I want to be off on my own. I'm going to get out of Epworth and be on my own. You know, the reason I say that, I've been asked time and time again by the staff here at Epworth, 'Man, you're doing so dang good. Why don't you just get discharged? You get the heck out of here.' I say, 'I'll tell you why, cause I'm not ready. And I lie in bed. I've had several staff stop me and ask me why I don't get discharged. It's because I'm not ready. As far as me getting back out on my own right now, I have one chance in ten thousand of being able to live on my own.

(snip)

L: Okay. But when will you know you're ready?

Richard: When, I think, I think when I know I'm ready is when I get, when I get out on my own. But the thing about getting out on my own, I feel like I'm not ready to right now.

L: But in what area?

Richard: Uh, the area that I don't think—is not being motivated enough. And by God, I'll get out? Like I got to be at work at 8:30 and here it is 8:15 and something like that which I know like here's what I'm supposed to give 6 hours, I give 5. I'm going to get a long talk. And—cause that's one motivation right there that I think real strongly about. And I feel like I don't walk like some little people do—I'm not talking about head injured, I'm talking about several other people, whatever. I'm glad I can walk out of here. But that's one of the things I have to live with. The other way that I know that I'm talking about is if I'm going to get out on my own and just forget this place. As far as me leaving here, say, the hell with you all, Dr. Rutledge, no way! You know what? Hell, I've been here too damn long. I went the long, long way and as far as me having to come back, I want to work in something but I could come back because I have the money. I'm guaranteed the rest of life, money due to my accident.

L: So, you're saying that you just want the freedom to kind of try your wings, so to speak.

Paula: He wants to be comfortable. That would be me. I'm not comfortable. I know, like he said, I can't...

Richard: But as far as me getting discharged and you not, I do. But I want to say that, I say, 'okay, I get discharged tomorrow. The doctor lets me go and says, hey buddy, you're on your own.' Okay. I get out on my own and in 4 or 5 days, everything is going to run amuck.

Terri: Something that's important to me is that—what I would like to do is get, is get out. Still be a client here at the program but get out and live in an apartment and see if I can do it. See if I can pay the bills. See if I can live on my own and have Epworth as a back up.

L: So, have a safety net.

Ellis: That's what I mean.

Terri: Yes, yes! But I feel I can do this and I don't feel that I am being given the chance.

L: Okay. That's fair enough. All right, so, you want to kind of just—you want to just test the waters.

Terri: Right.

Paula: I don't have a clue if I were to do that.

Richard: So, we're still going to do the same thing. You know, come on Saturday.

Ellis: I hate structure all the time.

As illustrated in the above discussion, the two-edged sword of rehabilitation structure, daily routine, cuts at the very heart of each survivor. It is critical to the survivor of a brain injury that he/she have a structure of daily activities in order to facilitate his/her progress. This structure provides the foundation for organization in daily living that is nearly always missing after a

TBI. It appears that individuals with TBI without some form of structure of daily activities struggle to mount any sustained momentum because they become easily side-tracked on purpose. The structure of schedule assists in identifying deficits, such as short-term memory of events, and offers stability within which to begin learning compensatory strategies to overcome the deficits. For example, the routine of daily activities following like structure each day lessens the complexity of events and allows the individual to concentrate upon memory pegs to retrain short-term memory. On the flip side of the benefits of daily structure, the repetition itself often becomes a source of irritation to the survivor over the years.

Learning Experiences

When I inquired of the clients how they moved from one level or stage of recovery to the next, they had definite ideas on the formula for improvement. Timing, mistakes, and individual styles of learning were three keys named by the majority of the clients. Chip offered these thoughts:

> Chip: Well, I think it will depend on the type of injury. I mean, some individuals can't remember anything for five seconds after. So, I mean, if you're telling them what the problems are, if they have a, like absolutely no short-term memory, they will just go in there and that's real frustrating to both—the individual and the therapist themselves. And I think that not always, it's perplex. I mean, because some people acquire knowledge through watching others without directly interacting between them. And I think the reason why that happens is cause they're afraid to display behavior or act, or appear that they will do wrong—display the wrong behavior. Then, you get your people that are basically sheltered.

> L: Okay. So, you think some people improve just by rote or just by doing something all over. They don't really understand why they're doing it. Is that what you're saying?

Chip: Well, it's kind of like getting on a computer. You need to know how to turn it on and how to access stuff. I think it's the ways in which people learn. Some people learn by watching others do it and others learn from doing it themselves time and time again, the repetitiveness.

L: Okay. So, you don't think that acceptance in your own self has anything really to do with it. Or it's not critical to it, I guess I should say.

Chip: I think it's important to make the individual feel comfortable and move at their own pace and not rush the program cause when you try to rush somebody through like a 6 month period or a 3 month period of time. Then you're going to miss out on the steps that are required for a successful transition. And you want to just basically make the client feel as comfortable as you can cause he's in a strange environment and atmosphere. I think that's important to make the client feel as comfortable as possible. And not so much give him everything but just outline what he can look forward to. And let him know the individual steps that he has to obtain these. Tutoring them is always good. Making sure they're orientated and knowing the rules and everything.

L: Good point about not pushing them.

Joe: It works for some people but some people can't hack it.

L: Uh-huh.

Chip: It's kind of like sending something UPS and they're on strike and you mailed it yesterday and it takes three days. And three days to send it and you mailed it yesterday, but they go on strike tomorrow.

Questions were often asked in conversations that indicated individuals' growing efforts as they were gaining skills that would be needed at their next level of recovery. For example, the following conversation illustrates how Todd asked not only of a definition for one word, retain, but the continuing conversation triggered another word, diluted, that Todd attempted to relate mentally yet was unclear of its definition. Not having been able to determine a definition during the context of the conversation, Todd had enough confidence in his mentor the

Clinical Director, Henry, that he asked this second definition although it was not in the direct conversation. Not to get sidetracked in this section on the issue of TBI individual/mentor trust relationship which is discussed in another section, but note the continuing conversation that allowed Henry to explain a bit more to Todd. These "teaching moments" were often overlooked by rehabilitation workers and in so doing, some of the gems of opportunity for both individuals' growth were lost.

> Henry: I was going to mention about the DDAVP. And that they'd cut you off one....

> Todd: Yeah. At lunch.

> Henry: I noticed your salt was a little bit low—your sodium was a little low.

> Todd: Cause I was putting out too much? That's when my salt gets low.

> Henry: In lower concentration means you're retaining fluid.

> Todd: I was holding too much fluid.

> Henry: So, that means your body's holding—and that's what the DDAVP does. It retains body fluids.

> Todd: It gets rid of how much—it keeps inside you how much your body needs and you get rid of...

> Henry: If you get the right dosage.

> Todd: Yeah. If it gets rid—it puts out, like disposes what your body does and doesn't need.

> Henry: No, that's not what DDAVP does. DDAVP only retains fluid. It's the hormone to retain fluid. It doesn't put anything out, your body does that naturally.

Todd: Yeah, I know. But it helps control on how much you put out, you know, like...

Henry: No, it helps control how much you retain. It's important....

Todd: What does retain mean?

Henry: You hold—the water you hold in your body.

Todd: Well, that's kind of what I was getting at.

Henry: No, it's the opposite of what I was saying. The way you said it was the exact opposite. It doesn't control what you put out. It controls how much you keep in.

Todd: If I wasn't taking this DDAVP, I'd be—I'd die cause my body would go dry.

Henry: Okay. Maybe. We're not sure, first of all that you need it.

Todd: All the doctors I've seen back home say that that's my most desperate medication.

Henry: Yeah. I believe you.

Todd: I just know that I've been told by medical doctors....

Henry: Sometimes things get better and in your case, you need less chemical. So, maybe your body on its own is retaining some fluid. I'm not convinced it's not. Does that make sense to you?

Todd: Sorta kinda maybe.

Henry: So, just like everything else. At times even hormonal function gets better just like behavior gets better. Just a process of healing and time. I'm not saying that's true. I'm saying we want to be very, very careful about this. You're right. If you do not have this hormone, you will pee out all your fluids and you could die. It doesn't happen very often because....

Todd: Diluted. What does diluted mean?

Henry: It means it's not as concentrated. It's not in concentrated form. It's kind of like the salt in your body. Think about it this way. You've got a certain amount of salt in your body.

Todd: Yeah. I need a certain amount..

Henry: Say, you've got a pint of salt. You got this much salt in your body [gestures to glass of drink he is holding] except it's white now, if I put this in a gallon of water, I have this much salt in a gallon of water. Well, say I give you DDAVP. All of a sudden your body is holding two gallons of water. Well, is this the same concentration?

Todd: No.

Henry: No, because it's diluted by two gallons of water, so your salt level would be lower. And that's what's happening to you right now. You may have the same amount of salt in your body, this much. But you've got two more gallons to deal with. So, you have a lower concentration. You have a more diluted salt content. Okay? I know it's a little hard to understand but just stick with me. Okay?

Todd: Yeah.

Henry: The body works in funny ways.

Todd: Yeah, I know it does. (laughs) it's too funny.

Henry: But, there's good news here, Todd. And that's that you're needing less chemical at this point in time. That's not a bad thing; that's a good thing. So, hopefully your body is taking into account that function.

The above conversation between Henry and Todd illustrates not only the value of client/mentor relationships and questions, but also the value of timing in a situation. One of the refreshing avenues to gaining momentum is asking a question. If the rehabilitation worker overlooks clients' questions or hastily answers, momentum can be stifled because it is a link to so many qualities for the individual such as perception of self, value, and achievement.

Just as timing and asking questions are important, mistakes are also great teachers. Richard had a knack for grabbing the essence of any situation and reducing it effectively to a few words. His reply to "talk to me about mistakes" was power packed in just three words: "Learn from mistakes." Individuals in both the facilities agreed that the freedom to make mistakes was an important learning experience:

> Todd: [Failure is important] because if you're given a task to do and you mess it up big time to where nothing can be done with it, next time they give it to you, you know you have to be more careful and not do it the way you did the first time because you ruined. So, you try to do it—you keep trying at what you failed and you try harder and harder and you're more careful at what you're doing.

In a conversation with several clients the value of mistakes was being discussed and suddenly the path of conversation took an interesting turn. The complex nature of motivational factors that influence an individual recovering from TBI is illustrated in this passage:

> Todd: Mistakes—like—teach the staff.
>
> L: What would you teach the staff?
>
> Richard: …to compliment them on their good points even if it's a small achievement. Compliment them a great deal so they will understand. Appreciate. They are good things and they not complete failure.
>
> L: Good!
>
> Myrtle: Tell you you're not a failure even though you have a head injury.
>
> L: Okay. They're not a failure even if they have a head injury. Okay. That there is something they can do? Is there anything they should not do?

Todd: Yeah. Definitely! I know exactly.

L: What?

Todd: [Expletives deleted] just like one of the staff here today. [Expletive deleted]sits there and he runs his mouth. He's putting you down in almost every word he says. He is putting you down, putting you down. "Oh, you don't want to do this cause you don't want to do this and you don't care."(mimics staffer) And he's ragging you out. He's not complimenting you at all. He's—more, he's putting you down more than anything else he's doing.

L: Okay.

Richard: He is the real tool. He has the head injury. He is [expletive deleted] himself. He is used to losing a great deal and wants other people to fall down to his level.

I heard the above conversation multiple times, just different individuals. I always sought to redirect such conversations to avoid client agitation. I generally directed it in the way of the value of our mistakes.

L: At the point where you are now, do you think it's important for you to experience failure just a little bit in order to experience more success?

Joe: Yes.

L: Why?

Joe: Be able to learn more. Be able to learn how to do things, able to learn how to do something but without having to be so worried—you know —you don't get in trouble

L: Okay.

Chip: Well, I think yes because failure is part of success. Before you can succeed, you fail at it once or twice before.

L: Okay.

Chip: It's kind of like riding a bike. You don't start off on two wheels. You start off on four wheels, then you go to three, then, you go to two.

L: Okay. So, you're thinking that failure is a foundation stone for success.

Chip: Yeah. It gives you something to build on. And to improve on and then reflect upon your failures in order to make sure that you know that they're still there and they can easily be reached back. And you can start all over again but that it—failure is a good thing cause it allows you to see how far you've come and then go farther and farther each time you fail.

The clients of the Tallangatta program were more inclined to speak in terms of the length of time required for recovery when discussing the movement from one level or stage to the next. These clients often spoke of their recovery journey. In the two examples that follow, the sections italicized indicate the manner in which clients would often refer to their progress through the stages of recovery. The italicized words indicate the phraseology most often used by clients in speaking of progress.

Tim: *I would tell them about how I was before I got hurt* and what I went through in the last 3, 4 or 5 years on being head injured. And I've been in there for a while, I couldn't even move, I couldn't walk and there always had to be someone there with me helping me and, of course, *I didn't know what the heck was going on.* I could care less. (snip). *I went* from being almost dead *to* up here where I have people come to me and ask me questions on my health. And in general how that makes me feel is very good. (snip)
. . .but it's going to take a lot of time. And when I say it's going to take time—like around years, they say next week… The hell with it.

Or Terri's interpretation: "Yeah, things are apparent to everyone else and the people are not putting you down. They're trying to help you see these differences. *And the best thing is just time.* I know that I keep repeating myself but *a brain injury takes a long,* long time to recover from. It's not just an overnight thing."

Assessment of Progress

The final subcategory of stages of recovery was that of assessment. The individuals in this study felt strongly that their ability to assess their progress along the way and see some positive results was critical to their ability to progress in rehabilitation. It was interesting to note the value of their assessment at the two facilities. Windy Hill, whose clients, with the exception of two, fell into the second stage of recovery, expressed the value of seeing accomplishment quickly. For example, time after time when Stan and I were working in the nursery together, and he was given a choice of chores, he chose the more difficult chore of sifting soil over watering the plants. When I asked him why, he replied, "It has a definite beginning and end. I can see my accomplishment and feel good that I've completed a job."

By the time the individuals had earned a move to the Tallangatta program, they vocalized the need not only for the assessment by those currently working with them, but those who had not seen them for a period of time. In addition to this feedback, these individuals were unanimous in their desire to test their skills in "the real world" without constant supervision.

In the following snippets from a conversation with Ray and Cecilia note, in the italicized statements, the way they continually compared their abilities to those of non-injured people.

> Ray: The thing is, the thing that's difficult, very difficult for me to grasp and hold on to is like I—*immediately after I got out of acute care, and immediately, I have to get back to classes.* I go into lecture halls and the professor would come in and lecture for an hour and maybe go to the board—good lecture, you know. And *I take notes, very thorough notes* and I would go out and as soon as the door would close behind me to the

lecture hall, I could look at my notes and they would make no sense to me at all. None! None! And so, and then see, that is what my life had been to that point. I was, if you will for lack of a better term, I was a professional student. And that's all that I did. And in a sense that's what I did. *And that's all that I knew. And I couldn't do it any more.* I had to drop back ten yards and punt. I had to do something and I... I... I...(long pause)

L: Go ahead.

Ray: it's just I didn't know. So, *I thought I'd just do something else.* I'll do something else. And so, I started taking a—I went to a school counselor and told him that *I wanted to do this and this and this.* He said, 'Whoa, wait a second! Why don't you do this and see how that works.' I ended up taking 22 preparations in restaurant management and PE and PE and PE...

Cecilia: And then *you get to where like you've got this feeling you're lost* and then, I come here. *I was about to go to college but I decided my life— I wanted to make myself happy—this happy thing. Not make myself miserable.* You know I was teaching which was a great art—kids. And then I came here and I really feel like what he's saying because you come here [state] and you're like, "okay, I'm going to come here and I'm going to be able to live and learn how to better take care of myself. And I guess people would make me perfect, sort of." But, and then, like I'm here 2 years and you're here 11 years. *And you're like, well, isn't it time I'm ready to go?* Aren't I—to get what I want? And, but what you want, if you're like me, what you believe you want doesn't change. I believe I want to go to college like all of my peers. *You believe, and I can rationalize the whole thing to death and understand that I have a brain injury. I can understand rationally but...(long pause)*

L: Operationally, it's hard, is what you're saying.

Cecilia: Yeah, it is hard...very hard.

As clients move from one stage to another, they often encounter the shock as Terri did, of not really knowing what to expect in her 'recovered world.'

Terri: Yeah. Because I noticed that when I went out on my home visit, that I was scared. There were times when I was like, 'What now? How do I react? Okay, well.' There's a fine line and that line here is, 'okay, I've

225

always got someone there saying, now, don't do this, don't do that. Now stand here. No. No. No.' and then, on my home visit, it was like, 'Sure, whatever you want.' And I'm thinking, 'Whatever I want?' well, what do I want? I don't know what I want because it's been so long since I was given that opportunity that, shoot, I have no idea. So, then I sat there like for a long time going and muddled over, 'What do I want?'

Thus, these three elements: (1) perception of recovery at any given time, (2) learning experiences, and (3) assessment of progress were all stimuli for the movement between stages in recovery. Individuals could cycle back and forth between Stage 2 and Stage 3 for an indefinite period, and then, one day, the momentum generated ultimately carried them to the final stage—progress enough to regain life back out in the community whether in a supported environment or in an independent living situation.

Achievement

As noted in Chapter 2, studies of motivation are often based upon the subjects' speed and ability in accomplishing a task with correlations being drawn to their motivation to achieve that particular task. Achievement of individual goals was rewarded at Epworth through means such as the token economy, the color system, and daily IBP (Individual Behavior Plan) successes. While individual response to these techniques are discussed in this section, it was the internalized effect upon the individual that placed achievement into the contextual category of perception of recovery. In the normal population, achievement studies measure the feeling of satisfaction upon reaching a specific goal and the energy created within the individual to repeat that success euphoria. In the population of the individuals with TBI, the energy created within upon achievement was more complex.

When individuals suffer TBI, they are stripped of their identity. Suddenly the person is fighting for life itself and once he or she is medically stable, the more difficult fight often is just beginning. As illustrated in the previous discussion of self-perception, the TBI individual looks in the mirror and sees someone who looks the same, but who does not act the same. The person can't explain his/her thinking, actions, or feelings. The individual with TBI is stripped of his/her social identity. Simple things that are taken for granted by most people are no longer properties of the individual with TBI. The items we often carry on our person such as keys, cigarettes, make-up, money, nail-clippers, and coins are no longer in their possession. Oddly enough, these physical objects help give us an identity. What the individual recovering from a TBI achieves then, the manifestation of that achievement, such as money, cigarettes, snacks, is only a small part of the energy created within. For individuals with TBI, the real motivator from achievement is not the accomplishment nor even feeling of pride in the accomplishment itself, but rather the regaining of a tiny piece of themselves. As the individual achieves, he/she gains ground in self-perception, which in turn yields productivity in his/her perception of recovery progress, and that generates additional progress, which ultimately elevates the individual to the next level. Obviously, I do not propose that this happened every single time, but rather it was this pattern that was seen repeatedly in this study. Isolated examples illustrate the energy and philosophy of positive self-images built when an individual with TBI achieved.

Example 1:

For Joe, the shift in self-esteem was strictly a mental thing, "It depends on how bad you want it."

Joe: To be able to fix a problem, you must be able to know how to do it first. Some people can wish all they want to and never get better. You have to want to get better. If you don't want to get better, then, there's no use trying. But some people have the tendency not to try and rather be a vegetable for their lives of their own will. (snip) It depends on how bad you want it. You want it badly enough, you'll get it. You'll just find a way to get it.

Example 2:

For EC, it was competing "...with the public...some of the big boys."

EC: Well, (laughs) I mean, what really as they say encouraged me to know was whenever I got to actually competing with the public. And some of the, as they say, big runners. Some of the, some of the big boys. And Hal, hum, I'm trying to remember how many years ago it was. It was about 4 years ago, 3 or 4 years ago, he told me, he says, if you get to placing in some of these area runs, then, I'll give you some more freedom and kind of like give you your own—kind of like let you train yourself. And so, at any rate, I can't remember exactly what year it was, but it was something like about '93 or '94, I placed second over here in the 'Run for your Life 5K.' And then, I turned around and actually wound up winning it one year. (snip)

L: Okay, so for you that competition and being able to be out with the big names and the other boys, was a critical factor in your knowing you were kind of back in the real world?

EC: I mean, it's, well, okay, let's do some, as they say, some storytelling so to speak, or imagining. Okay, you happen to have a head injury and you're a real good runner. You run 5K in say, for instance, 23 minutes. Well, I come out here. I've had a head injury. I'm approximately twice your age and I run it in 22 or in other words. And I actually go ahead and beat you. To me, that gives me incentive.

L: Okay. Why does that give you incentive?

228

EC: Well, okay, I know that you have the—I can see that you have the ability to be a top runner. But you, to give you an example, you push it too fast at first. And then, you don't hold enough for the end. So, that way, you've not got enough kick at the end and that's where the finish line is. And that is actually where the trophies are—is at the end, not at the first.

L: So, what you're telling me then is part of the way that you kind of knew you were really recovering and getting better is that you could, you begin to see yourself back into society competing. You are as valuable and important and as a whole person—your self concept changed. You didn't as much see yourself as head injured at that point as you saw yourself as a good runner.

EC: As a good runner and even a helper and a teacher, so to speak.

Example 3:

For Joye it was simply more individualized time with others, relationships, "one-on-one is a big-time motivator."

Joye   …one-on-one is also a big time motivator. If you came up to me and said—and you and I were buds, you say, 'okay, Joye if you get 100% in IBP this week, you and I can go out and catch a movie, grab a burger and then come to my house and we'll just veg for a while.' That's a big-time motivator! Relationships are what make the IBPs successful most of the time because, sometimes I look at my IBP like I don't care. It's not important, the relationship is.

There were times when the interpretation of achievement differed in the minds of individuals with TBI and their support and rehabilitation workers. This eroded the building of positive self-perception. Individuals, then, became less motivated to continue to pursue goals simply through confusion. In a group discussion, I asked the question, "On a scale of 1 – 10, 1 being the day of your injury and 10 being your return to whatever community and style of life you choose, where are you now?" Each of the three respondents offered a different self-evaluation:

229

Darrell: 9 1/2

L: 9 1/2? Good! Ernest?

Ernest: I'd say 10.

L: Ten, okay. Then why are you still here?

Ernest: It's...

L: You opened the door for that question.

Ernest: Okay, it's—I've always been really kind of hesitant about that because, it's a thing between my wife and I and it's more because she thinks that I'm just not completely working. And I think I've displayed enough of independence for 8 years.

L: Okay. How could you, then—what do you think you need to do in order to show her that independence?

Ernest: Take a—I guess take the steps to find an outpatient program at home and start working towards my goals. Goals for my job opportunity.

L: Okay. What's keeping you from that? Why don't you do it? It sounds good. Why don't you do it?

Ernest: My—I guess my idea of it is, I'm always—I guess I'm starting to look at that. He's thinking, too, that, Dr. Rutledge decides—when I say that and I put it like that, he says, well, whatever Dr. Rutledge says.

L: Darrell, how are you going to get from a 9 1/2 to a 10?

Darrell: Achieve. Follow through with my ideas and don't back down. Cause backing down all the time, is going to get you run over.

L: Okay.

Darrell: Each time you step backwards, there's always people higher up than you who have more authority than you who can knock you out of the ballpark. So, you've got to work with them so you can get over that hill, that hump.

L: Good! How are you going to get, Hugh , from a 7.5 to a 10?

Hugh: Well, let me fill you in, okay? The reason I put myself at a 7.5 is first off, I'm my own guardian. Okay. And I can leave. But I have no place to go and again, I procrastinate a lot on this and I don't look. And that's why I just keep staying here. And I don't know if I need to stay here and work on me, or if I need to look for some place to stay so I can leave.

The true goal of extrinsic rewards in this population was to create enough successes to build self-esteem while shaping a behavior. The hope was that self-esteem would overtake the drive for extrinsic reward. The individual at this point was making great strides in regaining control over his life. This is expressed by Chip in the following statement:

Chip: I think that if you gain satisfaction through completion of a task, then, I think that that's a little better treat to have than being motivated by money cause—I mean, money is a good motivator, but you should display behaviors for their own rewards—intrinsic motivation. Because in the long run, it will get you a lot more, I mean. Now, if someone offers you some money for doing a job, that's okay. But I don't think you should expect it every time cause you're doing this behavior to help out basically. And, if you get something in turn, that's fine and if you don't, that's fine, too.

Gauntlets: Motivators and Demotivators:

According to Merriam-Webster's Collegiate Dictionary, a gauntlet is "a long line of guards or well-wishers." To the individual recovering from TBI, the daily path to the future looks exactly like a gauntlet, lined on the one side with guards or demotivators and on the other with well-wishers or motivators. It is this subcategory that would most closely align itself with the traditional studies of motivation conducted over the last century. As introduced in Chapter 2, "motivation is the concept we use when we describe the forces acting on or within an organism to initiate and direct behavior" (Petri, 1991, p. 3). The two

231

properties assigned to this subcategory are motivators and demotivators. The total immersion I experienced as a researcher allowed me to watch these motivators and demotivators at work. The outcome of each event defined the path for the continuation of the day's activities. Each day from wake-up until bedtime was a gauntlet to be run by individuals in rehabilitation situations. I lost count of the times I saw individuals stumble along the gauntlet of the day, become demotivated, and struggle or become non-productive the remainder of the day. On the other hand, I also saw the reverse. An individual headed down the gauntlet stumbled and a staffer or fellow client boosted his/her spirits by some act seen as a motivator to the individual, and the entire course of the day was altered in a positive manner. The individual with TBI just needed to remember that we build or rebuild lives one day at a time. Twenty-one sorts of examples were offered by clients of motivators/demotivators. Eleven of these 21 were staff related, 7 being demotivators. The individual's job satisfaction and relationships with family and friends were likewise offered as both motivators and demotivators. The token economy system of gaining positive feedback and encouragement was by far the favorite motivator. For ease of grasping the essence of these data, I will illustrate the motivators and demotivators in terms of their common properties: personal, staff, and support.

Personal

Society tends to link our "selves" with our professional lives, our vocations. For the individual with a severe TBI, work usually is out of the question. For the mild or moderate injury, there may be struggles at work with executive skills that interfere with the productivity of the individual. Both types of injury were represented in the Epworth network client work force, both those working in the community as well as those working in a network-owned business.

"What doesn't work for me is adversive conditions, negative comments, feeling like the job doesn't matter, being depressed, and not liking the job," voiced Chip who worked in one of the network businesses. Individuals needed to feel their efforts were important, not just "busy work." Individuals could feel unfulfilled or became disgruntled at work yet had difficulty in verbalizing the actual problem, as illustrated in Cecilia's comments: "…One thing I would like is, is, I would like is, I, to be working and at the Buckeye [Epworth facility], I'm not working. Things aren't working. And they're not working, I mean…" As I watched Cecilia's momentum over the next few weeks, it seemed to drop to slow gear when time for work arrived, or when work discussions were present. Unfortunately, Cecilia was not able to pull together the necessary skills for work outside the network-owned facilities and the fact that her work was a demotivator posed a possible hindrance to further success.

Just as our work can demotivate us, it can rejuvenate our energies and put us on top of the world, as evidenced by snippets of Terri's conversation with Inez, the case manager for Epworth, after a few days at her community job. While this entry is lengthy, I think it bears consideration, for it is a very good example of the subtle changes momentum offers to self-perception and ultimately recovery.

Inez: Well, tell me about Little Italy. I want to hear about that.

Terri: Oh. It is going better than I hoped. I mean…
Inez: I hear you're money bags.

Terri: (laughs) well, let's see. Let me flip back here to my finance section [in daily planner] and I'm doing so well, I—my tip section on my first day, I made $8.29, and on my second day, I made $20.71.

Inez: That's wonderful!

Terri: Now, okay, I want you to know something. On Fridays that's a given because Friday in a college town, everybody wants pizza. I don't know what it is.

Inez: But you have to work harder for it, too. More customers! (snip) Yes, well they're supposed to tip. Not everyone understands the tipping process...(all laugh) Bet you understand it a lot more now! Right?

Terri: Oh, yes I do! And so, it's not a matter of—it's not free money. It definitely is not free money because we're making sure that—I mean, we wait. (snip)

Inez: How many hours do you have next week at Little Italy?

Terri: Uh, let me look. Okay, um, I don't have my schedule for next week.

Inez: yeah, you do, 12/15?

Terri: Oh, yeah, I do. I'm sorry. I thought that was like this past week.

Inez: Today is the 13th.

Terri: Okay. So, let's see—10 to 5 Monday and Tuesday, and then Wednesday, I'll be working at The High Road—my norm schedule. And then 10 to 6 on Thursday, 9 to 5 on Friday and 9 to 5 on Saturday. My supervisor is so wonderful. I was ready—my manager at Little Italy—she, I told her, I didn't even ask. I said, 'Well, I want you to know that I already have plane tickets and reservations to leave for my Christmas vacation. But I want you to know that this job is more important to me—starting and getting the feel of it and getting, that I will cancel my vacation and work here. And she goes, 'No, you take your vacation.'

Inez: What a great thing for you to do. You handled that very well.
Terri: Thank you but I was shocked, I mean, I was, I had made up my mind that this was more important. (snip) So, I mean I work. I mean, I get

up there and it's not—even when, this is a thank you to Epworth. And that is, when there's down time, like in between— when I've waited on all my tables and I don't have anything to do, I can roll silverware, I can clean up the floor, I can help wipe down the back counter area and kind of prep it. And when people are clearing off tables, go ahead—even when I'm not taking their tips, I can go ahead and help them out for when they're backed up. (snip) …it was just really neat and the fact that I wasn't scared or that I would just shut myself off. That I just opened up and said, 'Hey, yeah, well, this and this and this and this.' And I didn't overdo it.

Inez: Good. That's great. You know I think this is interesting reading your PIC [Personal Information Coordinator report] because all of us would look at your three weeks and say your biggest accomplishment is your job at Little Italy. You know what the first two accomplishments are she has down here for you?

Terri: Well, let me look. Let me think. My first two accomplishments would be, I would say, arrangements—that was….

Inez: More flexible in the program and improved interaction. I think that's very telling in three weeks. That's wonderful.

Terri: Cause at dinner at night when I come home from work, I'm just all bubbly and talkative and before…

Inez: On a natural high.

Terri: …well, before I would just sit there and eat. And I'd have people go, 'So, Terri, how was your day?' Same! No expression. (laughs) and now, I'm just like, 'oh, and this happened and this and oh, please, you know what? They have such attitudes. And these girls, they just gave me a great tip! And oh, and oh, and on and on.' And I'm kind of people are thinking—the dinner talk at night. I need to watch that.

The changes in Terri could be seen not only in her language and reports of the events and projections of the coming week's work, but also in her facial expression, and general non-verbal communication. She felt better within herself, her value as a person had increased in her mind.

Other personal motivators reported by many are represented well in this conversation with Chip and Joe:

Joe: Outings, staff, rewarding clients—that motivates me. Making it work, reinforces by token money and I have enough token money to buy things and you may have given me a reward for something. Plus, what I get now will help me eventually in terms of the things I want. For instance, I need like money, cigarettes and stuff. That's what motivates me.

L: Why does an outing motivate you?

Joe: Because it gets you out of the structure [daily routine of rehabilitation network].

L: Okay. Gets you out of the structure.

Joe: That's the last thing I enjoy is time out. Sometimes, we even go to the town and have a nice couple of hours. It's never that nice. Something to do.

L: Okay. Is it because it's in town and away from the structure?

Joe: That's part of it.

L: Do you get tired of the structure?

Joe: Yeah. I do get tired of the structure sometimes.

L: Okay.

Joe: And sometimes when you do nothing that's actually beneficial like stay up late or some of the snack time or soda, that's good. It shows that you're positive inside. Makes you feel happy.

L: Okay. Chip, what works for you?

Chip: Okay. Uh…

L: I know cigarettes work for you. What else?

Chip: Not necessarily. I just smoke just because I can. I mean, I've gone a week, two weeks without a cigarette and…

L: Okay. Good! So, you're not hooked on them, in other words.

Chip: I am sort of but, it's not. I can go without. I mean.

L: Good! I'm glad to hear that.

Chip: I think the biggest motivator for me is freedom. I mean, trying to do what I need to do in order to have greater freedom both in Epworth and eventually outside Epworth. And, being by myself is also another motivator. I like working by myself. I like positive reinforcement, satisfaction, job completion, liking the job, stress—believe it or not, I work best when I'm under stress, time frame nearing an end.

Freedom, an interesting concept. Each of us desires the freedom to be ourselves and be valued for it. The individual with TBI is no different. Recall the self-determination theory of Deci and Ryan (1991): an individual wants to be in control of his/her life.

Staff

Without a doubt, those working with an individual with TBI were in a precarious position. Often to assist the individual toward recovery, they had to be stern. This sternness was sometimes misinterpreted, and at other times was not merited at all. Part of that dilemma lay in interpretation. Nonetheless, the staff interactions with rehabilitation clients held a large key to the individual's future, for often the recovering TBI person was like an empty page waiting for the mentor to write the story, a new beginning, a second chance at life. All comments regarding the staff, whether they were as demotivators or motivators revolved around two themes: time and the value of the individual.

1. <u>Time</u>. The lack of staff time to just listen and hear what the individual was saying was a major demotivator to clients. Clark challenged those in charge to,

> listen, because it might not be important to you. But it's important to me (snip) I mean I've had a lot of things that I've asked for which were important to me but weren't important to [staff names]. And, it really hurt my feelings. I really got hurt....that—to us, we're here to learn again over and over. But that's not helping by telling us no or not doing what we ask. Or they say one thing, and then, just cutting off the rope or something, you know."

EC illustrated a frustration of short time for guidance,

> ...lots of time not saying that my opinion or my idea is good, but it's inside of me and I want to talk to someone. ...but there's nobody here to talk to because you done walked off. You told me, "hey, later." What later? You're too busy...Okay, you go an hour or two later, what in thunder was it that was so important. Well, I can't remember. It wasn't that — and it's not that your memory's that bad in one respect, it's that, well what was it we were talking about? Downright frustrating and irritating it is.

On the other hand, the time and care were also valued by individuals, as Terri expressed of staffers attending her while she was in the hospital,

> ...is when I realized when I went to the hospital and when I woke up or became aware of my situation. Here I am in a hospital and I look to my right and see Glenda and I look to my left and there's Bess and I'm thinking, 'these people care. I'm not just a buck! I'm not just a way for them to earn money. They've been here in the hospital. I'm here and they care about me.' And they sat there and they held my hand when I was scared and they helped me. And I felt like a person. And I just, I felt encouraged to trust.

2. <u>Value</u>. Resentment toward the staff built when the individual with TBI did not feel valued as a person, a human being. From the long-term clients like Ruth, "Hot shot staff that don't know what they're talking about when they are

giving you direction" to the new clients like Wally, "staffers tell you different things, who do they think they are"; each had an opinion, an individual interpretation of his/her perception of staff interactions.

One interesting common point of view of the clients at both the Windy Hill and Tallangatta programs was the difference in the sympathetic and empathetic approaches attempted by the staff. For example, one Sunday night a group of us were just sitting and chatting after a semi-structured interview. The guys had come to like the Sunday night group sessions and did not mind "going on record" with their opinions of all sorts of topics of their choice. Pet peeves was the topic and Darrell's voice raised sharply when he declared, "It kind of gets me upset a lot of times that people see me like this. And you always hear, 'I know what you feel like.' No, no you don't know what I feel like. You ain't been through this from 23 to 37. Don't give me that BS." Often, staff were so eager to show their concern and understanding, it was misinterpreted by the clients. Because the individual with TBI had lost his/her own perception of self and was struggling to reconstruct his/her own life, he/she was slow to trust others for fear of being hurt. This tentative time of building trust, then, caused some communication problems for the staff/client relationship, when staff attempted to respond empathetically rather than sympathetically. In every walk of life, it is difficult without "walking a mile in the other man's shoes" totally to feel and understand what a person is going through. The TBI population was no different but perhaps was more sensitive to their comrades and to those not in their inner circle of experience, due to the fact that they were dealing with the brain, the very center of one's "being-ness."

239

The best of intentions can be seen on the part of the staff and the height of individual interpretations, albeit perhaps incorrect, of the clients:

Cecilia: I'll spit it out. I hate the phrase always used, "Get in trouble" and stuff like that is just like I—how people do not grow up. They, go in the meeting like I won't grow up. Like I'm scared to accept responsibility for myself. And then, us "get in trouble." Well, I'm willing to accept responsibility and learn. Then I'm not scared to "get in trouble" cause it's not trouble any more. So learning is another way to open my mind. And as far as, like one thing that really, just 'f_ _ _ you' is sort of my state of mind, is staff—client relations. I was at a place (snip) that they weren't staff and clients. They were—(laughs) it was emotional. Therapeutic rehabilitation center and it was a school and we called the teachers by their names and they called us by our names. They were teachers. This staff shit just, in my mind says they're better than me. 'I'm better than you.' And because I have this title I'm better than you. Now, the word Doctor, comes in different. If you're in medical, yeah, they probably have more information than you and about one certain thing, but...still I have to live with the brain injury so I still know some things...

L: Okay. That's fair enough.

Cecilia: One thing! One thing that bugs—okay, there's one person here—there's some staff here that we call clients behind their back. When I get shitty, I call them client. 'oh, you're just a new client.'

L: I hate to think what you say about me behind my back.

(laughter and Hugh says: Oh!)

Cecilia: And everyone—and they're supposed to be there to help me?
L: That's fair enough. What about you guys? (snip)

Hugh: Now, saying, 'okay, you have a head injury.' And it's easier to be around you because you've been there and we can say things around you that say, with Thad and we're talking about that—oh, you shouldn't talk like that, you know. Just say, no swearing or whatever. And he's got a higher age on us and he can put us down. And just because of that; just because he works here. He's a staff, you know. And where a patient or whatever, he's just trying to say, you shouldn't say this or this or this. You know, trying to help us or whatever and—well, just like me and Ray , this friend of mine, we can talk about this and it's okay. Some people you can't do that with. Like I said…(snip) Now, the other clients or me, say, either that's not right for staff to do that to him, they see the light.

L: Does that help you, though? Does that help ease that pain back down?

Hugh: Not right away. But it does inside. Inside my head, I think 'oh, great. I'm glad you know.' They feel the same way I do.

L: Ray, what is your response to that?

Ray: Yeah. The thing is like it would be an ideal situation if it worked. That we didn't have a stratified system, but it is, must do this, must do that—a necessary evil because—and the specifics are very blurred but I think that we need to change our terminology about "getting in trouble." Because I think that like it takes everybody—like I'm sure everyone is working together. If you take a look of the situation of, well, there's staff here and there's clients here, you know. You just have to look it as, I am here and everyone here is working to become a better unit rather than competition these people are already better and these people aren't as good. And these people are trying to help these people because you'll "get in trouble" doing that.

Hugh: If you have a group like—have a group of clients here and a group of staff here and you know both groups. And you come into which group you want to go to, I'd pick the clients group. Okay? Because, I mean, they think more like you because they're like you in a way.

L: That's fair enough.

Hugh: I mean you can say, wow, they're great. There's nothing wrong with them. Wrong! And these guys will—okay, we're all clients. We all think pretty much the same, you know. And have the reasons why we need to get out, you know. Or do what we need to do.

The other common area of complaints rendered about the staff was that of

interpretation of events:

Cecilia: Oh, yeah, she [staffer Edith], I mean, yeah, I mean like she was being demanding. And then I was—she called it, 'being unflexible.' I said to be very unflexible. And that's right, that is right, that is right. That's right actually. That's right. Um, now that I remember that in my

241

restatement, speaking, I realize that right like, but not then, she said, 'Go ahead and do it, maybe you and Paula can work on it—together you can work on it. You know, she can tell you. You can work together—this and that.' And I was in no real inkling of a space to want to work with Paula , to work, to deal with her, to deal with her. And then, we ended up doing some working—it wasn't really together, now and then. And I was like, 'okay' you know. And I was like, 'This is cool. You know I can be more flexible. I'll take it personally. I'll deal with it on my own. I'll deal with this. I'll be more flexible.' And then, again, I felt I was pulling a lot of weight still when we were working together. And she told me what was wrong with me, er, not, yeah, what's wrong with me and how I can do it better—I can be doing better. And let's just get this done. I've got so much to do. And I was trying, at that point, I was trying to be a friend going, 'Listen! You are going, you know how you tell me when I'm going fast. Well, that's what you're doing.' She's like, 'I've just got to get things done, da, da, da, da, da.' Like, 'okay, forget it! Forget—I could use a profanity—I was like, why? Why am I—she's not listening to me basically and then at the end, I ended up being the one who—I mean two different times At the end, I ended up, I ended up putting something up and Edith says, 'Well, weren't you all doing this together?' I go, I go, well I was just putting up the mop bucket. Like I took up for both of us and Edith never saw what really happened.

Misinterpretations also occur when the client and staffer disagree on the events that have occurred. This is no different from any other relationship of leader and follower such as employer/employee, professor/student, parent/child; however the misunderstanding can be exacerbated because the client has suffered TBI and is already struggling with communication matters.

Ernest: "It kind of makes me mad when the staff, they talk to you like you're confused and you don't, like you don't know nothing. You're confused and you're brain injured. It just makes you mad. (another person says uh-huh.) you, too? I mean you forget stuff every once in awhile but when they act like you're brain injured and you'll—you're confused. You know what I'm talking about?

Darrell: I know exactly what you're talking about.

L: Give me a specific example, can you?

242

Ernest: Okay. I say about 3 or 4 years ago the staff members—and some of them's still around today, you know. When I was in this program for about 6 months, you know, most of the staff would just come in my face and say, 'well, you said you did this. You said you did that. You didn't do it. You ain't got it in your notebook. Go outside. You're confused.' And I would really get so puzzled in my mind that I'd say, 'what was I thinking?' You're confused! They're the ones that are damned confused. And I would stop myself before I would start going—cause I like to go on and on and on. And most—come my injury, I have that to where now I can slow myself down a lot more kind of talking that way because I don't want to get excited and get agitated to where I start getting mad.

In one informal session, the consensus of group opinion created this charge to staff: "Show me you know me over and over and then show me you support me, have listened to me before you stereotyped the behavior, because over time I can change and may not be the same person you keep thinking you see. Listen to me. Put your feelings at your job, not just your intellect."

Support

The overwhelming motivator for individuals to gain enough ground to be discharged from the rehabilitation network was to return to their own community and be with or near family and friends. If the individual did not have the infrastructure of family and friends for support, his/her rehabilitation momentum could be diminished.

VISION

"As a man thinketh in his heart, so is he." (Proverbs 23:7) In every walk of life there seems to be agreement that the thoughts, the visions, of an individual largely direct his/her paths and achievements. If one does not aim, surely he/she will

243

miss the mark. Our thoughts, our visions become our goals. The analogies offered in life for goal-setting are bountiful: goals are like our road map on the highways, our navigational instruments in the air, our lighthouse upon the sea, our blueprint for building success, our score for the symphony, the target for our arrow, and so forth. In classrooms across our land, teachers assist students in setting goals, "reaching for the stars," achieving their best. I doubt that there is a coach, at any level of a competitive event who does not set goals for his/her athletes, urging them to "see" themselves upon the winners' dais. As discussed in Chapter 2, the self-efficacy of individuals was often correlated to the level of goals they set for themselves. The higher the self-efficacy, the greater the goal. Also noted in the review of literature, the goal level did not necessarily correlate to the accomplishment or effectiveness of the goal. The vision for each individual with TBI needed to be cultivated and defended individually. No support members, nor caregivers, nor friends could do it for her. This category emerged mostly from field data, observations, just watching the phenomenon happen time and again over nine months. I divided this category into three subcategories: goals, God, and hope/humor as shown in Figure 5.6.

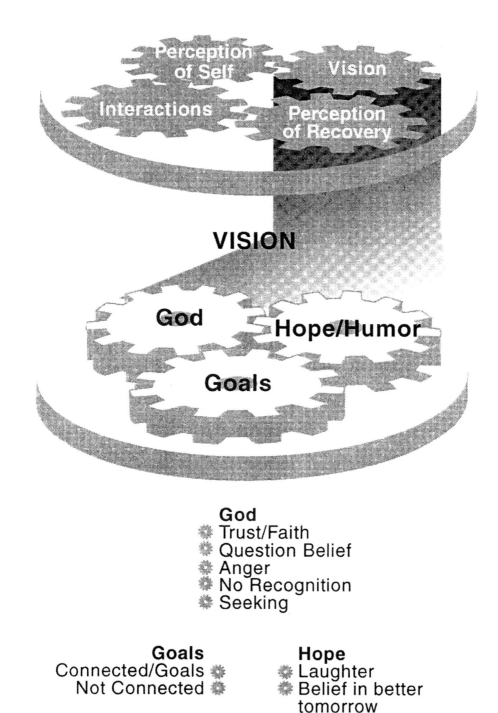

God
* Trust/Faith
* Question Belief
* Anger
* No Recognition
* Seeking

Goals
Connected/Goals *
Not Connected *

Hope
* Laughter
* Belief in better
tomorrow

Figure 5.6.   Contextual category: Vision

245

Goals

From my observational notes, it appeared that individuals whose self-efficacy was higher also had different visions of their goals, of what would happen to them in the future. In the TBI population observed in this study, individuals who possessed a strong sense of self-efficacy appeared to behave in a more resilient way, that is, they could bounce back from minor misfortunes of their rehabilitation efforts more quickly than individuals with poor self-efficacy. This resilience was made possible for these individuals because of the complexity and multitude of motivational factors present in any category.

In general conversation as well as in semi-structured interviews, I often asked the question, "Can you see yourself being discharged from Epworth?" I received a variety of answers: "Not really," (Myrtle) "I, yes, I can see myself getting home…it might be, uh, two or three years, but I have patience" (Richard). "Definitely." "Umm, yeah, if I keep doing what I'm doing" (Todd). "I wish" (Ray). "Nope, no place to go" (Ruth). "When I'm ready" (Darrell). "Would like to but probably not, 'cuz I have plenty of insurance for the rest of my life so I'm not gonna be discharged anytime soon, no matter how good I am" (Tim). "My folks want me here" (Hugh). "Good question" (Stan). The individuals who answered in a negative or doubtful manner always seemed to drift through the day. As I repeated the question at different times during my months of observation, clients often answered differently at different times. Their perception of discharge potential usually matched the type of day or week they had experienced. The individuals who were able to imagine discharge, though they experienced troubles, often rebounded from struggles quicker than those who had no picture of leaving the rehabilitation center.

Another way I enjoyed testing their "vision" was to ask the question, "Where are you on a scale of 1 – 10, 1 being the day of your injury and 10 being discharge back to your community to resume life the way you wish." The individuals answering in the doubtful or negative category regarding "visualizing their discharge" often gave me a score of 3.5-6.0 on the scale. Those who could imagine the future outside of a rehabilitation center usually offered a rating of 7-8. Finally those with definite goals or plans, such as community college, or GED work, or some vocational job such as grocery sacker, or fast-food host/hostess usually gave a personal rating of 8.5-9.5. I can not explain why, but these ratings, unlike the question, "do you see yourself discharged?" did not vary from one time until the next when asked.

I spent a tremendous amount of time (easily over 150 hours) working with Myrtle. Recall Myrtle replied, "not really" on some occasions to the query, "Do you see yourself discharged?" Myrtle was a good example of those who fluctuated in their assessment of discharge potential. On days when I focused my attention to working with Myrtle on ways her activities helped her to get better and one step closer to her goal of taking care of her toddler daughter, she was most energetic and enthusiastic during the day. For example, when doing floor exercises during physical education time, I challenged her with questions such as "How many do you think your daughter could do?" or "Explain to me how to do this exercise as you would explain it to your daughter." When working on her speech projection abilities, we would often play the football cheering game she would one day teach her daughter when it came time for her daughter to try out for cheerleader. I had Myrtle stand yards away from me and lead the cheer, "Give me an F" and I'd reply "F"; "Give me a R" and I'd reply "R" and so forth until we had spelled a name of another of the clients. Then she would conclude the cheer, "Fred, Fred he's our man, if he can't do it Greg can…Greg, Greg he's our man, if he can't do it…" and so forth. Not once in all the months I worked with Myrtle did she ever ask to stop any of our "games"; she was content to work for long stretches. Of course, the longest stretch without a break of some sort was only 20 or 30 minutes. In the early days of her residence, we sought to teach her the daily schedule, or structure as it is called at Epworth. Her attention span was minimal as was her concentration and her frustration tolerance was extremely low, which would trigger a cursing streak that could make even a sailor blush. As the days grew into weeks and then months, as the staff learned more about her just by listening and incorporated those ideas into her daily activities, she began to blossom albeit at a low functioning level due to her injury. The magic? There was none, but rather I believe it was the environment and the multiple sources of stimuli given to Myrtle. The stimuli, focus upon Myrtle's interests, and time were the ingredients to aiding Myrtle. Days when she replied negatively regarding her image of discharge were days when I could track activities that had somehow failed to bring Myrtle's goal, her daughter, into the picture. This was true even in light of difficult times. For example, cursing was tamed in part by asking "Would you allow your daughter to do this?"

The argument may be made that the value of working with the goals of an individual with extremely limited short-term memory and a poor medical prognosis was counter-productive because those goals will, in all likelihood, never be met. After watching even the small differences it made in the happiness and self-esteem of an individual, I ask "Why not?" Who are we, the caregivers, to say what will and what will not happen? In Myrtle's case, chances are she will never be independent, much less capable of caring for a child; however, time will take care of that issue. If we, at this point, can assist her to put forth her best efforts in rehabilitation efforts now, perhaps we can assist her in achieving a better future, limited though it may be. Myrtle was not an isolated case in observation; I saw this phenomenon of rehabilitation efforts rejuvenated time and again when related to the clients' personal perception of the future.

One of my most encouraging cases of seeing this phenomenon of vision work was that of Stan. Prior to his accident, Stan had been a successful university student. Stan did not suffer from a lack of confidence. He did suffer from a lack of awareness of his deficits, or at least seemed to. Stan was the one who boldly announced that he had not accepted his injury in order to protect his ego. I spent close to 200 hours with Stan and during that time, he taught me a great deal. His long-term memory and incredible gift for words, spelling, grammar, general knowledge was still intact. His short-term memory was weak and he was physically limited by the left-sided hemiparesis resulting in unsteady gait and upper body tremors. His medical prognosis was bleak when it came to the probability of independent living and likewise to gainful employment. However, Stan did not see it this way. As I began to watch the interactions of Stan and various staff and note our own interactions, I noticed there seemed to be "spurts" of his ability to remember short-term items. He had what I call a "TBI selective memory." When something was important enough to him, he could remember it. As I watched over the weeks, his stated goals to me never changed; he wanted to perform. Reality said he probably never would attain his goals but who is to say? Actors suffering from Down's syndrome are getting parts in made-for-television movies. Christopher Reeve has brought world-wide recognition to the productive lives of spinal cord injury survivors and need for further research of spinal cord injuries with his television appearances. Why not an actor who has suffered TBI?

Another interesting way of studying the goal-setting abilities of these individuals was in the discussion of future time perspective (FTP). Nuttin & Lens(1985), noted that FTP is the theoretical bridge between motivation and volition. That is, FTP connects the thinking about goals to the initiation of processes to achieve those goals. According to Nuttin and Lens (1985), FTP refers to "temporally localized [goal] objects.... that occupy [an individual's] mind in a certain situation" (p. 21).

As noted in Chapter 4, I administered a future time perspective questionnaire to participants. While the findings, at this stage are inconclusive, the data raised several interesting areas of thought regarding the influence of a link to the future and goal setting for individuals with TBI. As I mentally compared the story of Stan above to the experiences I had with another client, Todd, I noted several interesting issues raised in the variance of methodological procedures employed. On selected items for comparison, these two young men had similar quantitative FTP scores on the questionnaire and their overall scores were similar. However, the scores failed to capture the qualitative differences in their future time perspective obvious to me from my informed insight. I offer several differences for the discrepancies between these data. The participant may offer responses they view as socially desirable. Upon first glance, their item responses appeared to be congruent with their interview responses. Both are similar in the "amount of connectedness" and "value" reported; therefore, both Stan and Todd appear to share the same amount of future time perspective. However, from my observational notes as well as interview data, Stan provided a much more detailed description of the future and his mental links between the future and the present. While I believe that FTP knowledge can be of value in the rehabilitative process, several additional problems arise in this quantification of FTP. To what extent is the participant's response to the questionnaire a function of time spent in the rehabilitation facility, to the time post-injury, or to the individual's stage of recovery? Are clients less likely to feel connected to the future in a residence setting that is removed from "real life"? Furthermore, to what extent is FTP related to the type and severity of head injury? In the case of Stan and Todd, Stan suffered a much more severe injury than did Todd; therefore, he has great difficulty in follow-through of his ideas and goals, which hampers his being able to gain momentum from his connectedness to the future.

Rehabilitation caregivers must channel these links to the future and aspirations into functional, practical rehabilitation efforts without destroying a dream in the process. This was certainly easier said than done. Often Stan began to perseverate upon his goal and did not connect to the tasks at hand. While that is a critical issue in the rehabilitation efforts, that is not the argument at this point. The argument for this subcategory is that the image individuals hold for their futures, however great or small, whether their goals be 15 minutes until the next cup of coffee or 15 years until the starring role on Broadway, that image affects their momentum of progress. This image then is critical in the motivational picture of rehabilitation. As was the case with Myrtle, when Stan's rehabilitation efforts were presented as stepping stones to his ultimate goal, he performed and progressed at a better rate.

I remember the advice given by Dr. Rutledge at a staff meeting regarding one individual's inability to see a future, "He's got a little bitty world. Let's stay inside of it. If we stay outside, we lose him. If we stay inside, he has a great life. Remember, he has never had a date, never had a close friend, never had a wife, never had children, and never will. Stay in his world." This individual's world, his future, was generally what was about to happen within the next 30 minutes or had happened within the last 30 minutes. As long as he was spoken to within that window of 30 minutes either side of reality, or elected some topic from his vast background knowledge, such as the world wars, he was happy and enjoying life at his level of ability. Certainly for most of us that lifestyle would not offer happiness, but the quality of life is defined from within the one who is living that life. We cannot define the future nor happiness for any individual.

God

The second subcategory of Vision is that of faith, a belief in God. Again the majority of this interpretation is from field notes. The impact of a spiritual base was certainly not difficult to see in clients day in and day out. Perhaps my favorite thought from a client with regard to God came in a conversation with Ruth. Ruth, a long-term resident, and I hail from the same home town and that

252

fact was the foundation for the friendship that we shared. Ruth has been through a lot over the years having had a successful marriage, professional career, and active social calendar prior to her injury. Ruth was extremely slow to trust and to share, so I felt honored that she took me into her confidence and shared her ideas and opinions with me. After we had been chatting awhile, she reminded me several times to be sure and share with people to "…appreciate life and live it to the fullest. If I'd known what was about to happen I'd sure have appreciated things more. I went from all to nothing in a car wreck. I was just living a normal life, a normal life…" Her voice trailed off as she obviously was traveling back in time in memory of better days, when suddenly she looked at me, laughed and said, "Look at me now, I've made it, I've regained a pretty good life. I wonder what God thought when I was told I'd never amount to anything. We got the last laugh."

Unfortunately, I have no record of the author of the next story, for the story was jotted down quickly in my field book. I had been assigned "church duty" one Sunday morning, meaning that I had the privilege of being one of the staff that accompanied the clients to the community church service. This particular week, it was the local Christian Church. Following the service, we were standing around talking and one of the Tallangatta clients drew a cross on my bulletin and said, as he drew the vertical line, " I like coming to church because if I'm connected vertically" and then drew the horizontal line, "I can make it horizontally." In our discussion that followed, this client explained that when he felt connected to God ("vertically") his daily life ("horizontally") was easier. He explained that the inner peace that he felt when he was "listening to the

Holy Spirit" helped him make choices and overcome the hurts of his daily life. I glanced again at the cross he had drawn as I placed the document in my field books. How true, I thought.

Many clients expressed the very same words as Fred "just to know that God kept me alive for some reason helps me look forward." Often I noted that clients would retreat to their rooms when angered and read their Bible, a calming effect. Clients often related their strength to their spiritual ties as Cecilia did, "...I believe that Jesus is with me. He knows what's right in my mind. He—what is that word?—subject of His?—[Holy Spirit was client's reference] what humans can't be. I mean, if He was here. I listen to Him and trust Him ...somehow, spirituality has been my only motivation."

Other clients recognized the value of spirituality in their peers, "...but I know with Ronnie, Ellis, and Don, church is a big thing. So, if you could have some sort of individual religious time set aside for just them and you—individual time."

The clients at all Epworth facilities have the opportunity to attend church if they wish. During my days at Windy Hill, a representative of the Catholic church came to the facility and conducted a brief service with several clients who were unable to attend the weekly mass. This practice allowed the clients unable to attend to have spiritual contact and partake of communion. To my knowledge, all the clients with whom I worked were of the Judeo-Christian faith. The subcategory of God is not intended to suggest one religion over another, rather it is intended to make the observation that a spiritual foundation and practice in the lives of the clients did affect their momentum during the day. Clients with some religious belief and/or affiliation seemed to be more content, more easily calmed in crisis, and more resilient in their troubles. I noticed less anger and bitterness in these clients. I believe that spiritual freedom, which cannot be taken away from an individual, gives any life meaning and purpose.

Hope/Humor

The final subcategory of Vision is that of hope and humor. Hope is the inner warmth people feel when they eagerly anticipate with confidence some coming event. For the individual surviving TBI, hope is critical. The individual must see some glimmer of better days ahead in order to overcome the devastating loss of self. The loss of hope and courage can have a devastating effect upon an individual suffering from TBI. There is a close connection between the state of mind of an individual, his/her courage and hope or lack of them, and the state of immunity from crisis his/her body will understand (Frankl, 1984).

Coupled with the element of hope, the individual in crisis needs to be able to laugh. It has been well documented that humor can lift one above adversity and push him/her toward survival in the worst of conditions. Humans have an internal instinct to fight for self-preservation, and humor is one of our best tools. Clients often commented on the lack of humor they saw in the staffers, "They never laugh," (Richard); "They get nervous if we horse around, I wanna shout loosen up, give me a break!" (Tim); "Her sense of humor lacks two things: sense, and humor." (Ellis). The esprit de corps that was evident at meal clean-up or group outings seemed to be directly related to the staffer in charge and the amount of freedom the clients had to clown, laugh, and just enjoy life.

255

One of the most enlightening statements I heard during my nine months at the Epworth facilities was offered by Hugh, "We've gotta be allowed to enjoy the here and now, not always be geared for the future for this is our life right now. I would relax a bit and have more fun in the real world, I want to do that here also—I don't want to live like I'm at summer camp all the time."

INTERACTION

"Different people in different positions at different moments will live in different realities" (Shotter, 1993, p. 17). Shotter noted that there is a special knowledge each of us must acquire, "how to be a person of this or that particular kind according to the culture into which one develops as a child" (1993, p. 19). This knowledge, continued Schotter, is the kind of knowledge one has from within a situation, a group, a social institution, or society. A portion of the difficulty for TBI clients is dealing with the intertextuality, already formulated knowledge, of the group in which they reside post-injury. Whether it be the home, rehabilitation, community, or work environment, chances are the individual with TBI will struggle partly because he/she now has lost some of the skills of how to act in those "realities." The greater the memory loss, the greater the potential for interaction difficulties. As discussed in Chapter 2, we are socially-constructed. The loss of the knowledge of one's social-construction will manifest itself differently according to the injury sustained. Whether the loss be great or small, the outcome is the same, strategies for interaction are weakened. There was no need for elaborate communication models to explain the difficulties. The simple model in Figure 5.7 indicates the five key areas for communication break-

down: sender, message, interference, receiver, feedback.

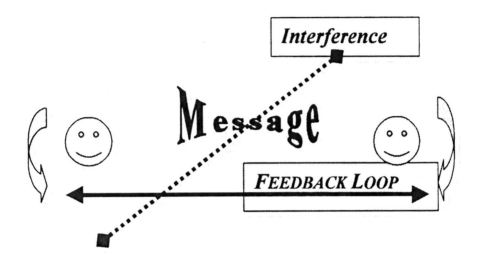

Figure 5.7.   Basic communication model

The communication breakdown can occur for any number of reasons, for

example: the client does not encode or decode the original message clearly;

he/she does not understand the message; interference of some kind, such as an

interruption, hinders his/her communication and/or concentration.

Four subcategories contained in the contextual category of interaction

emerged from data analysis: relationships, community, technology, and touch, as

represented in Figure 5.8.

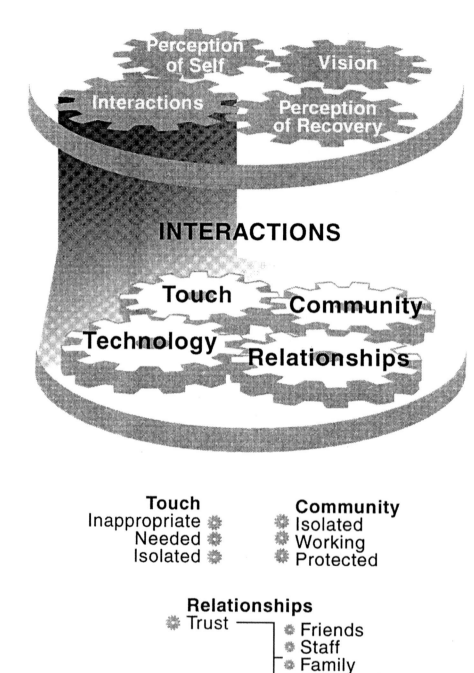

Figure 5.8.   Contextual category: Interactions

Relationships

Represented in this subcategory were all the support network members with whom an individual with TBI communicated on a regular basis, such as his/her medical teams, family, friends, co-workers, and fellow clients if in a rehabilitation situation. Because the primary properties for each of these relationships were the same, I offer the examples in light of the client and staff relationship. The interaction relationship bore three properties: trust, respect, negotiated meaning.

Trust

Imagine being 3 or 4 years old again and recall the security you felt in your parents' presence. You probably were slow to trust anyone outside the family circle of friends. You did not need to be worried for Mom and Dad were always there. Now imagine that you suddenly are rebuilding your life, possibly with large chunks missing from memory, or perhaps your long-term memory is fine but you are unsure of the proper routines for daily living and your intertextuality of values whispers, "trust family only." Now, compound that feeling with the frustrations of communication in general, words you no longer have at your fingertips, events, places that no longer fit into your schema of life. You are afraid to trust quickly. Trust must be built again, just as it was when you were a child, except now, you do not feel the same security blanket as before even though it may be present. For the individual with TBI, the sense of self and your new reality is perplexing to say the least.

Ray: …what is important in 2020 is that in 1998, I knew who I was because then I could get all that other stuff figured out. But if I don't know who I am precisely, then, it doesn't matter all that other stuff. If you decide, now, this would be good for you and this would be good for you, etc. and that's not what I think, why should I trust you?

Often clients became muddled in their thinking mixing "theories" or prior knowledge incorrectly. For example, Cecilia felt that money buys all sort of things and hence, noted a reason not to trust staff until she was absolutely sure that they were paid to "help" her:

Cecilia: I think I know the reason. I'd trust you quicker if you didn't charge me. If you were a rehabilitation place, and didn't charge money. Because I mean if I could—that's one of my cop outs—one of my back doors, cop outs. The reason not to work—I'm paying to be here and I rationally and intellectually want to understand, want to believe that you're here to help me and things like that. Number one I can go to rationalize things, I wish I was more aware of myself, like it's all the Mickey Mouse operational definition. "Will initiate client feedback to staff members and staff, da, da, da, da…." I don't understand. All I know is I'm a human. I'm a person with feelings and you're the doctor. This is where I come from usually. Or I usually come from, you're the doctor and just I don't trust you. First off I come here with loads of distrust of my own self, of other people and I cannot have a concrete answer—you touch me here and it's going to be better and it isn't. And, but so, if you didn't charge me money, I think I could very much learn to accept that I was here. But, I have a family who—outside, this is not my only reality. And it's very hard for me to live a reality as Ray is saying to begin with. To just live in reality of my certain situation. (snip) …to trust, it's really knowledge. I guess, knowledge because like a doctor—doctor, not Dr. Rutledge , but the neuropsychologist, or another, a medical doctor. I was not in this situation cause I don't trust all—cause he's under a contract and my total trust does not go to them because they've got all this system to answer to. But they have information that is concrete or precise.

We do not often calculate how much emphasis we place on "knowing" someone before we trust them. The same seemed to be true for TBI individuals. Len phrased it rather succinctly when answering what was the most difficult aspect in his entire rehabilitation program, "(pause) Having to take orders from people I don't even know."

Respect

Speaking on respect she felt she was given post-injury, one of the Preliminary Study 1 participants said, "Hey, I'm not stupid, I have a brain injury." Her statement has echoed in my head now over a year, so periodically I asked other brain injured individuals their response to the statement. Chip had an interesting reply:

> "It's a cop-out. Because what you're doing is you're saying, I'm different. Treat me differently where we're no different than anybody else. The only thing we have is we have a brain injury but that does not put us in a bracket by ourselves. We are still part of the human population. And should be treated and have everything that they have."

I often received the point of view from clients at both the Windy Hill and Tallangatta programs that they felt treated as "less that equal human beings" by others. When Ernest noted, "I get tired of people treating me like I don't know anything," his statement was met with resounding praise and agreement from all five clients in the group. The word "respect" was their choice to define their frustrations. Perhaps not as eloquently spoken, Todd expressed the same disappointment:

> "Like, just like, ever since I've been here [Epworth] when I was in [another rehab], I'd tell the workers over there, "Okay, I'm not capable of doing that because of such and such thing." And they said, you know, that's a good enough reason. And I'll do the same thing here or I'll say, "oh, I did that by accident. I didn't mean to break it." And the next thing is, "No, there ain't no accident." Or just like with my memory, just cause I don't have a memory deficit, I'm not allowed to forget nothing except a

lot of the staff here do and that OK. It's against my right. It's like, it's me creating the biggest crime on this planet if I forget something sometimes.

An individual's desire to be recognized as somebody of importance and value did not change simply because she had a brain injury. I do not propose that the viewpoint of the individual with a brain injury is always correct in his/her interpretation of receiving "no respect," but I do offer the proposition that it is his/her interpretation and by being such can create interaction problems if others are not sensitive to the possibility.

The position of participant-observer was a most interesting one considering the potential for bias to enter my research. As discussed previously, being aware of limitations that could be present in my viewpoint because of my own personal experiences, I took precautions to maintain such conflict at a minimum level. I am confident that I accomplished this, and I am equally confident that some of the insights emerging from this study were largely due to my experience and ability now to "see both sides." From my vantage point, respect was most interesting and painful to study. An unusual opportunity to see "both sides" occurred about three-quarters through the primary data gathering. I had been working at both the Windy Hill and Tallangatta programs by this time for months and was well known as the "staff/intern" by many. My personal TBI history was not known in detail by anyone and was known as a casual fact by many, more clients than staff. Because I kept regular staff hours, the fact that I was primarily a researcher faded in the background. An interesting turning point in this study came in late November when I experienced a partial seizure, which caused me to temporarily disassociate from the environment and forget the occurrence. No clients were present, but staff were aware of the incident. In the days and weeks that followed, I noticed some interesting differences in the manner in which I was treated. The staff were divided in three ways: some sought my opinion of "what's happening for so-and-so" now when a client encountered difficult times or there had been a communication breakdown; most treated me no differently; and the third group caught me by surprise—I felt like a client again. I felt "talked down to," I was "corrected" often on items that previously had progressed with no mention. For example, the manner in which I might instruct the client to put away the dishes in the kitchen, or the order I suggested that they prepare for arrangement meetings was questioned and I was asked for verification. I was asked, "Do you want to write this down to remember it?" when given instructions by some staff. Instructions that just the previous week those same staff had given and thought nothing of it because I was "staff," now were explained in detail as if I had no clue what to do. Suddenly, I felt that sick feeling I'd experienced so many times in the last decade, I had less value as a person, the mutual "human being respect" had vanished. The rest of this interesting story is that the clients, on the other hand, "closed ranks" and became very protective of me. They began to resent the manner in which I was treated and spoken to by certain staffers and voiced their opinions. Clients sought me out, wanting to talk about the frustrations trapped inside that they had trouble understanding. I certainly could not answer all their queries but it did offer a tremendous opportunity to study how and what generates the momentum for an individual with TBI.

The clients at Epworth all were trained in the skills of RBT, Rational Behavior Thinking. This program, originally designed by Maultsby and

Hendricks (1974) was used to teach the individuals that others could not control our feelings. The program taught individuals to think through a problem and analyze their feelings and deal with the real issues, not the superficial ones. Because I had experienced this program as part of my staff training in the early days of summer before this project began, I was able to use that experience as a teaching tool for the clients during these periods. For myself, however, the fact remains, that finding myself treated—or at least feeling that I was treated—in that "spoken down to" manner altered my own momentum. I am now far enough removed from some of the most painful rehabilitation days that I can cognitively create a rebound for my perception of self—in the early days, I could not. Many of the individuals with whom we worked were still in the "early days." Their rebounding ability was not yet developed and to sense you have no value or respect as a fellow human was disheartening.

Mutual communication

As discussed in Chapter 2, Wells defined negotiated meaning as "two or more people working together to resolve a problem by means of talking, thinking, and acting in collaboration" (1987, p. 3). This final property of relationships holds the key to these relationships. As suggested in the study of Holmes (1996), the patient/doctor relationship is based upon mutual understanding. An excellent portrayal of negotiated meaning at work in this population is offered by Todd. The following discussion is an excerpt from his Rutledge Day review meeting. I had been working with Todd during the prior month and had created for him large posters for his room to serve as memory pegs and posted check-points for reaching his ultimate goal, being in partnership with his uncle who was in the construction business. We worked for over a week practicing how he would present this material to Henry at the meeting. Todd was on a natural high the day of the meeting. I had attempted to install a bit of positive self-image for Todd by calling it his business—rehab was his business for right now and we could learn the construction business principles by applying them to his rehabilitation program. We had planned his speech and I encouraged him to be positive in his description to Henry, and at the conclusion of his discussion to invite Henry to be on his imaginary Board of Directors. All of our practice went down the drain when Todd arrived at the meeting and had difficulty in his new role. My heart sank for fear I had taken him too fast toward interjecting humor that might be misunderstood. At the infancy stage of visualizing his business, Todd did not have the communication skills to pull off the subtle humor. His social skills deficit allowed him to stumble in the gauntlet of the day. Fortunately for Todd, Henry quickly saw what was happening and allowed Todd to "play out his role." This situation was negotiated successfully because Todd trusted Henry and Henry respected Todd. Note the progression of Todd's gaining confidence in his program as he and Henry discussed it, then Todd carefully following our "plan" for his invitation; his tentative nature when at first the humor wasn't understood, and Henry replied in his administrative voice; and finally the beauty of negotiation, leaving room for respect of the individual with a TBI. We join the conversation after Todd's program and goals had all been explained and his charts had been displayed:

Henry: Well, I think it's a great idea. We'll see how it works.

265

Todd: I hope it works out now.

Henry: I think it has before.

Todd: It's a good program, I think.

Henry: Well, I think you'll enjoy it. I think they're some realistic goals.

Todd: Yeah.

Henry: Now, this will be over your bed? [referring to charts on display]

Todd: Well, this one right here will be beside my bed above my clock radio, my radio.

Henry: Accessible. It's got to be where you can write easily on it.

Todd: Yeah. It's—like my radio and clock is only, comes out about that far from the wall. So, I'm real capable of writing on it.

Henry: Excellent! No problem. Well, good luck.

Todd: Thank you.

Henry: I think this is a good plan.

Todd: No, we didn't put it above my radio, did we?

L: It's just on the wall, right there by your chair where you can get to it.

Todd: For the moment, it's there.

Henry: Well, we'll see how it works out. You'll know in a couple of weeks what revisions it needs.

Todd: Yeah. So, you want to be one of my associates. Well, not associates, what are they that you were saying, he was?

L: His board of directors—they give advice.

Todd: What?

L: Board of directors—they give advice to the company president.

Todd: Yeah. Would you like to be on my board of directors?

Henry: For?

Todd: this program?

Henry: Don't worry. I will be.

Todd: Well, I would like to see your job application.

Henry: I'll give you feedback on a consistent basis.

Todd: Yeah. I'd like to see a job application.

Henry: Well, I'm not interested then.

Todd: (Laughs.) Hey, come on now! You're getting into my business!

Henry: (Pause) Okay. What's in it for me?

Todd: To see how well I do.

Henry: Well, that's not enough! What's in it for me?

Todd: For you?

Henry: Yeah!

Todd: Seeing how well you've trained people to successfully work, help a client.

Henry: Well, I want something concrete. Ice cream, candy, you know, I can deal with that. Fruit, apples are my favorite.

Todd: You pay for it, we'll order it.

(laughter)

Henry: Well, you better figure out your reward system for your board of directors, there, Bud.

Todd: Hey, I don't make much token money, so…

Henry: (laughs) Well, if we have a board meeting where there are Twinkies out there, I'm ready to go.

Todd: Just as long as the…

Henry: As long as you're paying for it.

Todd: Just as long as Windy Hill is paying for these Twinkies.

Henry: No, man, you've got to make it worth my while.

(continue to joke)

Community

Whether it be school, church, social or sports club, or another organization, each of us feels a connection to some community outside our homes. When that connection is interrupted we feel a sense of loss that is often difficult to pinpoint. Returning to the communities of one's pre-injury self is difficult. High levels of anxiety arise due to problems caused by memory deficits, behavioral outbursts over which one has no control, inappropriate social skills. The individual with TBI can not explain why he/she act, thinks, walks different, it just happens and is frustrating. The embarrassment that can occur in public often deters some from attempting such a venture again. This fragile feeling in the community concerns individuals in the later stages of their rehabilitation:

> Terri: Hope that I'll find an answer. Hope that I'll find not just an answer to, 'Oh, well, yeah, I've got short-term memory loss.' But an answer, or answers to my questions as far as, okay, what kind of techniques could I come up with to make, to make what I am doing now not as difficult. And

how will I use that information out in the world? And see here, I'm so protected. I'm ostracized. I'm just completely removed.

L: From whom or what?

Terri: From public.

L: From public?

Terri: Because we don't interact with the public. We go and we sit down, we watch a movie. We go and we sit down and we eat dinner with ourselves, you know, in a protected atmosphere. But we don't have interactions with the public.

L: So, protection to you is a negative factor.

Terri: Yeah. Because I noticed that when I went out on my home visit, that I was scared. There were times when I was like, 'What now? How do I react? Okay, well.' There's a fine line and that line here is, 'okay, I've always got someone there saying, now, don't do this, don't do that. Now stand here. No. No. No.' and then, on my home visit, it was like, 'Sure, whatever you want.' And I'm thinking, 'Whatever I want?' well, what do I want? I don't know what I want because it's been so long since I was given that opportunity that, shoot, I have no idea. So, then I sat there like for a long time going and muddled over, 'What do I want?'

Therefore, whether or not the individual recovering from TBI feels

connected to the community does indeed become a factor in his/her self

perception and definition of his/her progress in the recovery process.

Technology

Data analysis showed that the subcategory of technology had two

properties: training and connectedness.

Training

There have been many empirical studies investigating the effectiveness of technology such as computer assisted instruction or video in rehabilitation programs for individuals suffering disability (Bloom, 1987; Brennan et. al, 1991; Brennan et. al, 1992; Deardorff, 1986; Graham & Schubert, 1985; Kim, 1995; Petzel, et. al, 1992; Skinner et. al, 1993) using technology. However, often left out of discussions in these research reports is the importance of instructor assistance. While the scope of this study did not include any direct evaluation of technology and its use by the TBI population, I did have opportunity to make two interesting observations.

First, because the most frequent ages of injury in the United States are 16 and 17, most TBI individuals have grown up enjoying all types of technology. Rebounding from TBI, the individuals who were able to use the computer exhibited a definite boost in their perception of self for they were "with the times." The computer became an ally for many who were severely handicapped like Kyle. Kyle had a sharp, quick-witted mind trapped inside a body that now did not serve him well due to his injury; however, he could communicate effectively via computer. Though the task was laborious and took a long time, Kyle was able to have contact with the world outside through the World Wide Web or Electronic mail (e-mail). I was amused on more than one occasion to have opportunity to watch Kyle and Richard work together on the computer. Richard was just learning to master the computer so he and Kyle often worked together as a team, Richard "dictating" to Kyle. Kyle often just silently corrected or altered Richard's words and kept typing.

Another young man, Neal, was not capable of using the computer at this point, but he recognized the "importance" of its power though he probably did not understand it fully. I attempted to see what would happen if I linked one very sharp computer client, Chip, with Neal to create a web page. Interesting journey! Chip appeared to have a sense of responsibility and importance because he was to design and create this web page. Chip and I discussed that Neal would not be able to understand all he was doing and that it was important to take him slowly. Chip labored on his questions for Neal striving to ask just the right questions. The frustrations came out in large quantity on this "experiment." On the one hand, to the extent he understood the concept, Neal was very excited about the web page and Chip was excited about building it. Chip did not possess a great "follow through" or stick-to-it-tiveness, therefore, I needed to hound him constantly to progress on the project. In addition to the client difficulties due to their injuries, we had network computer problems as well as arrangement struggles. I was combining young men to work together who were residents in two different facilities and meeting at a third facility to work together—but could only do so one certain day and time each week, and this added to the frustrations. However, in spite of the difficulties, during the times we actually were successful at getting the two together to sit before the computer and work, the self-perception level was visibly increased.

On yet another occasion I was able to provide a series, Brain Train (Falconer, 1996), for use at no cost to the facility classroom. This program had been designed specifically for use with the TBI population building cognitive and vocational skills. In spite of this gift to use, there was no staff in either of the two

271

facilities where I worked to provide instruction for the clients in order to make use of this tool. Therefore, while all the research projects can confirm hypotheses that "technology works," it is critical, especially in the TBI population, to have someone designated who is there to facilitate its working.

A second observation was the use of technology seemed to encourage the individual with TBI to feel connected to the "real world." Not only did the individual feel better about him/herself because he/she was "smart enough" to use modern technology, but also it allowed the individual to have contact with others through avenues, such as e-mail. There are listserv groups on the World Wide Web for special interest groups. The St. Johns' University maintains one for individuals who are survivors or connected to TBI in any way. Electronic friendships develop and events of daily life are shared. Within the Epworth experience, I had occasion to communicate regularly between universities with one client, Paula, who was enrolled as a college student in the local state university. At times on e-mail, we were just "fellow students" chatting about this test or assignment, and at other times Paula would send a plea for help or advice. It was a unique side of our relationship when I was at work, for we had our e-mail in common which silently "elevated" her for she had a piece of "technology" the others did not have.

The "technology booster" did not necessarily have to be a computer or television. It often was as simple as a fax machine. In a special project with Darrell, I arranged for him to fax me a daily report on days when I was not at work. This responsibility with "technology" elevated his feeling of pride in himself and his abilities. It was a joy to teach him what a fax machine was in the first place and how it differed from copy machines or computers and then to see the ease with which he carried out his responsibility. Darrell would often mention our "fax" communication in the presence of others, a sign that it did, indeed boost his perception of self.

Touch

Unfortunately, following TBI, individuals, especially young men, often have difficulty with sexual appropriateness. The hormonal imbalance overrides their better judgment. Therefore, many hours must be spent teaching the social skills of appropriate "touch" in public. However, human beings are born to crave the reassurance of love and affection through touch. There are times when just the reassuring hug is a boost to the individual with TBI. The tragedy of this vital teaching requirement is that it forces caregivers to walk a fine line between inappropriate behavior and the caring, reassuring touch.

The Interactional Strategies

It would be nice if the equation for motivation was simply, "S + C = O Stimulus plus Cognition equals Outcome" but it is not. According to Charlton (1987) one often may do something differently from what he wishes to do, sometimes even the opposite of personal wishes. This weakness of will, or "akrasia," suggests that our "…voluntary behavior itself is not the product of a simple, unified agent; but rather it is the emergent result of many competing intentions or wills" (Reed {1994} citing Holt {1915} in Neisser & Fivush).

Therefore, this complexity of internal drives and conflicts cannot be reduced to a few simple dichotomies, such as intrinsic or extrinsic motivation, or rational or irrational thinking patterns that seem to proliferate in the literature.

These data suggest, rather, that motivation is the by-product of a synergy, a momentum, created by complex interactions at multiple levels of specificity. As mentioned in the introductory notes of this chapter, the synergy of the motivational point to be made is illustrated by a gyroscope. Figure 5.9 illustrates the gyroscope analogy of motivation, generated by momentum. In order to portray the significance of the gyroscopic interactions, each part is defined, followed by the explanation of movement through case studies.

MECHANICS OF THE GYROSCOPE.

The heart of the gyroscope is the rotary disc (1), comprised of four compressed discs (2,3,4,5), representing the contextual categories. The rotation of each of the compressed discs is powered by interlocking cogs (Figure 5.10), representing the sub-categories of each contextual category. The rotary disc (1), representing momentum, is mounted on an axis (6), representing the antecedent condition of personal premorbid characteristics. The two axes perpendicular to each other and to the axis of spin represent the other antecedent conditions: personal support network (7), medical support (8) and manifestations of the injury (8). The weight (9) at the top of the primary axis assists in the balance of the gyroscope and is dependent upon enough torque to align the balance. This weight represents the core category common to all three studies, reconstructing self. The torque created by the rotary disc keeps the gyroscope moving. The rotary disc is free to rotate about one or both of the axes perpendicular to each other provided there is enough torque (10), representing engagement. The gyroscope is powered by a "power cord," (11) representing the energy generated from the interactional strategies. When the shaft direction has enough torque to stabilize its direction, the gyroscope can be gently maneuvered to another location, position, or inverted on its axis. If the gyroscope is moved abruptly, the torque is thrown off balance causing the gyroscope to stop. When the torque no longer is creating the angular momentum, and capable of withstanding the oppositional force, the gyroscope winds down and stops. What the model represents is that momentum (motivation) is to the TBI individual's rehabilitation engagement, hence progress and 'recovery,' as torque is to the balance of the gyroscope.

The challenge for the individual with TBI is to generate enough positive momentum to counter the oppositional pull from forces counter-productive to his/her rehabilitation program. These data suggest that within the four contextual categories interacting to generate the momentum, motivation, there are well over two dozen competing factors pulling for or against the individual's momentum. The "power cord" for one's momentum or motivation is the interactional strategies. The combinations of events in the four contextual categories yield the momentum for an individual. There are unlimited combinations that can serve as

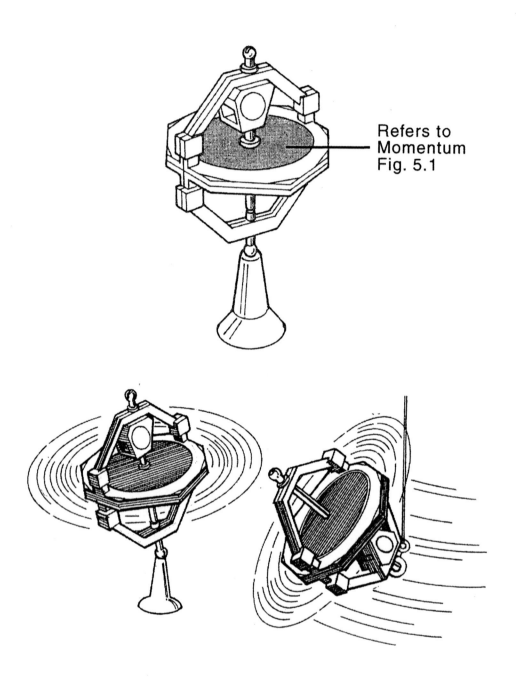

Refers to
Momentum
Fig. 5.1

Figure 5.9.   The synergy of momentum

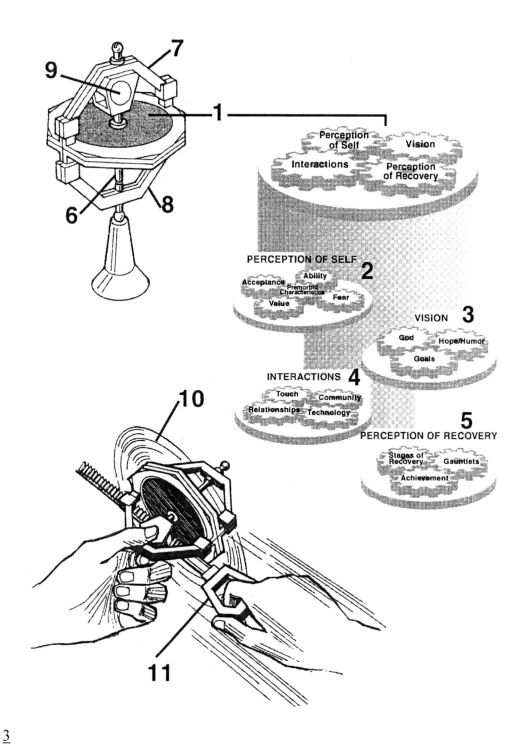

Perception of Self
Vision
Interactions
Perception of Recovery

PERCEPTION OF SELF **2**
Acceptance
Ability
Premorbid Characteristics
Value
Fear

VISION **3**
God
Hope/Humor
Goals

INTERACTIONS **4**
Touch
Community
Relationships
Technology

5
PERCEPTION OF RECOVERY
Stages of Recovery
Gauntlets
Achievement

<u>3</u>

<u>Figure 5.10</u>.   Mechanics of the synergy of momentum

277

the "power cord" to the rehabilitation gyroscope. The fine balance comes when the negative force(s), torque, are overcome by positive torque. The torque relationship is illustrated by the various interlocking cogs on each of the discs. If only one cog is moving counter-productively, the other cogs on the disc can still get the disc moving positively. Even if one or two of the disc are rotating negatively, the power of the other two may be strong enough to overcome the negative forces. This may occur in a brief span of time, fluctuate rapidly over time until it stabilizes one way or the other, or take long periods of time to occur. To summarize the gyroscopic relationships, four brief examples are presented from the data and illustrated with the gyroscope.

In the stories illustrated by Figures 5.11 and 5.12, an arrow followed by a number □1 indicates positive momentum, and an "x" followed by a number 62 indicates negative forces slowing the momentum. The numbers are sequential illustrating the flow of the momentum.

Todd's experience on one Rutledge Review Day illustrates that the synergy of momentum can be gained and lost all within a short period of time. (Figure 5.11) Todd was told in his meeting that he was being considered for a move to the Tallangatta program, a "rehabilitation promotion." In his contextual category of perception of recovery, he experienced a terrific boost. □1 He also experienced a boost in the area of the gauntlet for he had been paid high compliments by the staff. □2 This news, in turn, generated a greater self-perception for Todd. □3 The time of day was approximately 10:30 am. As Todd was celebrating in the dining area talking to fellow clients, Darren, a fellow client, gave Todd a slap on the back to which Todd flared and the two got into boisterous verbal warfare with increasing decibels. 64 About this time, Anna Ratchett (composite staff member) entered the room and demanded an explanation of Todd. 65 Todd replied, "If you don't move, like, the second he asks you, he puts his hands on you. And I don't like clients or even staff putting their hands on me for no reason." 66 Without asking Darren for any explanation and in front of all other clients, Staffer Ratchett chided Todd for his behavior and put him on time-out from the structure for the next 45 minutes to earn his way back for lunch. 67 By the time Todd reentered the structure, his vision of the future as a Tallangatta resident remained, □8 but had dimmed in its intensity, for in Todd's eyes, it sounded good but he perceived that he was not treated fairly 69 in Windy Hill, so why would a chance to move be any different. As positive as the future potential of a move and the present praise of staffers in his meeting, the hasty negative reaction by Staffer Ratchett stopped the building of momentum. The earlier positive forces did not give Todd the momentum, torque, for the day to overcome the counterforce, so Todd drifted through the day without making much progress. Staffer Ratchett entered notes at the end of the day, "Todd appears to be unmotivated today." 610 The next day's morning staff then read those words and already, the momentum Todd had to build had major forces working against it in potential staffer opinions. 611

The reverse effect is presented in Figure 5.12. Consider the last 24 hours of Ellis. Ellis was reminded to limit his weekly calls to 15 minutes each. □1 When one of the evening staffers returned to the office 45 minutes later, Ellis was still on the telephone. Knowing he had arranged for only two calls, the evening staffer requested that he hang up. 62 Following the conclusion of Ellis's phone

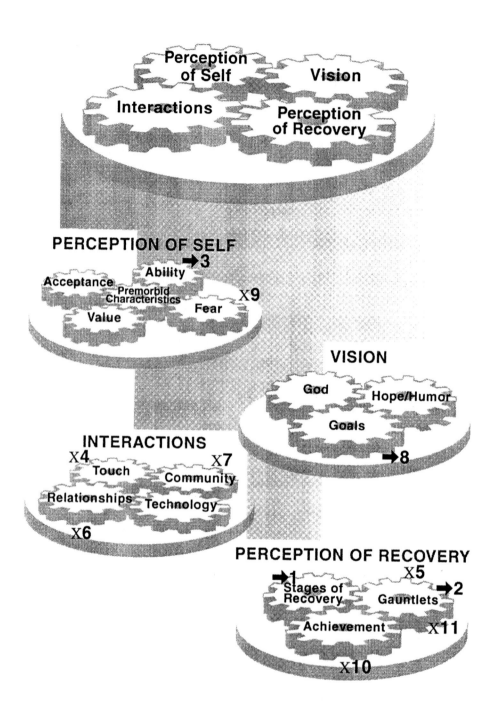

Figure 5.11. Todd: Rutledge review day experience

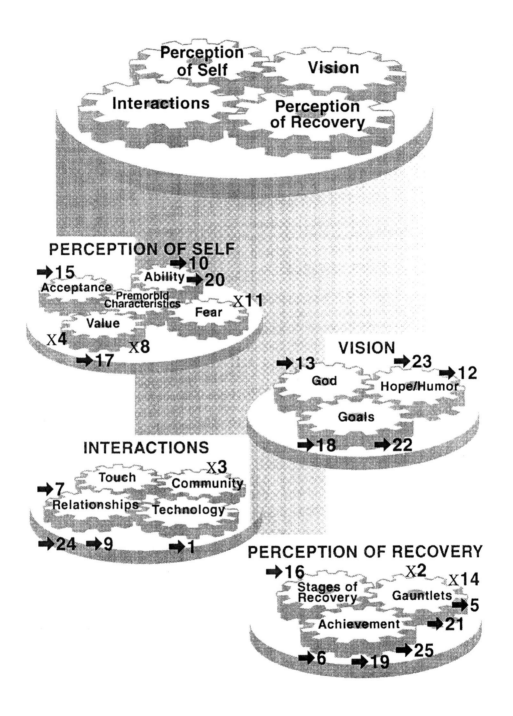

Figure 5.12.   Ellis: A day's changing momentum

281

calls, the staffer reminded him he was cheating himself as well as the other clients and staff by not following the rules. □3 This caused Ellis to feel a bit guilty, thus negatively affecting his self-perception for the evening. □4 Feeling down, Ellis headed for bed and called it a day. This evening staffer, Colton (composite staff), sat to enter comments in the log for the day. □5 His choice for entry on Ellis was a notation of his helpful nature on the afternoon outing and subsequent evening meal preparation. □6 No mention was made in the notes of the phone call. □7 Colton apparently felt the 15 minutes over time was not so important because it was the first time it had happened, and Ellis was talking with his parents and his former high school coach. The next morning, Ellis dragged into the breakfast area still feeling that twinge of remorse for the bad ending to the previous day. 68 The early morning staffer, having read the log notes for the day before, congratulated Ellis on his fine outing □9 and meal preparation assistance the day before □10. Ellis accepted the compliment but was puzzled because the phone call was still the key event from the previous day 611 that was on his mind since he hated to "get in trouble." Although Ellis's momentum was still primarily negative, the glimmer of a compliment at least shifted his thinking pattern momentarily. During meal clean-up, Ellis and fellow house residents enjoyed a few jokes and talked of the sports games of the weekend □12. Ellis told the joke he had heard at church the morning before and that positive feeling he had when he was at church flashed through his mind □13. Ellis nearly missed the van departure for work and was reminded that he needed to program his data watch if he were ever going to be successful 614. Though the comments regarding his tardiness were corrective in nature, Ellis had enjoyed a great morning with his housemates, and so he just laughed at the comments of the staffer □15 and did not let the complaint down his spirits. On the ride to work, Ellis's mind continued to role-play the compliment from the early morning staffer and his surprise □16. As Ellis contemplated the conversation, he decided that Colton must, in fact, value him as a person □17 and the contributions he made to write that in the log. It has now been 2 1/2 hours that Ellis had pondered the compliment. Ellis commented to me, "see Colton is different than Anna, he understands what is important in life and helps you reach your goals □18. I get so tired of Anna telling me, 'I know how to help you just listen to me.' What does she know, she's just impressed that she's staff and we're her subjects. I figured out the difference, she likes power, he likes me." Ellis's momentum was beginning to change. At work, Ellis successfully completed the tasks assigned □19 and admired his handiwork in the nursery □20. At lunch, the manager of the nursery told Ellis he had really improved in the organizational skills of his nursery duties □21. Ellis now was beginning to feel really good about his accomplishments and was beginning to imagine the next step in his rehabilitation process □22. Because Ellis was feeling better on the inside, he was beginning to produce more on the outside □23, which in turn generated more praise and positive interaction with staffers and fellow-clients □24. By mid-afternoon, Ellis was feeling on top of the world and working hard on his assigned rehabilitation duties □25. Several seemingly minor events, together, generated enough synergy in momentum to overcome the looming negative feelings. Ellis's gyroscope was finally balanced and spinning at top speed, at least for the time being.

Darrell is a good example of disappointment so deep-rooted from interactions that the climb for positive torque is made more difficult to obtain and retain. After many series of little disappointments, none appearing big at the time, along his rehabilitation journey, Darrell has developed an "on-guard" attitude.

> Darrell: Okay. A boxer has a coach. The coach gets the boxer all built up. But when it's time for the fight, the bell rings. The coach ain't there no more. Just the boxer. They don't know what they're out there for. And of course, then you're by yourself. So, what the hell do you do next?

> L: Okay. So, what you're saying is that the boxing coach is still on the sidelines.

> Darrell: They're not on the sidelines when the boxing coach—when they call, like call the people, who was there? He was always there. But sometimes, there's time when they teach them some stuff [on the sidelines]... It ain't hard. Go work on it. Cause I knew he wanted it. With all the roots—the long, long roots off of it. The thing about bonsai— I knew what he wanted. I say, 'what do you want?' He goes, 'I want this down—this or this.' I say, okay, work on it. You know, the coach. The boxer has a coach always on the sidelines. I'm tired of the coach not being there after the training to help me make that final step. I'm always seen as the old boxer, just learning...well, I ain't.

Because Darrell perceived that he was treated the same as in the early days of his rehabilitation and because he felt "left alone in the ring," it was more difficult to generate the momentum and sustain the positive progress that was a natural by-product of momentum. One could argue, "Well, that is ridiculous, Darrell has not advanced as far as he thinks..." Perhaps not, but as long as Darrell perceived the negative force(s) in his rehabilitation, the gyroscope will not spin freely propelling him to his victory of recovery—that is, his interpretation of a good quality of life.

The final example of the magic of the gyroscopic potential in the contextual categories is that of redirection. Just as the gyroscope can be gently redirected or even physically moved to another location while spinning, likewise can the individual with TBI be redirected. Stan was a model illustration of this phenomenon. Stan had the tendency to perseverate upon one or another of his momentum contextual categories until he appeared to be increasingly demotivated. If one could redirect Stan's negative force(s) of perseveration in one category and counter with strong positive force(s) from another category, then the negative feelings could be overcome, and though still present, momentum could occur in spite of the negative force. If the positive action could be sustained long enough, the negative factors would fade in importance and the individual would ultimately grow past this stumbling block in recovery.

Conclusion: The Storyline

Unfortunately, this story is repeated thousands of times each year. Without warning, a sudden event permanently alters the brain function of an individual. The medical advancements of the last decade have increased the number of brain injury survivors. For the individual with a traumatic brain injury, the ultimate recovery challenge—community reintegration—is enormous. An injury to the brain does not manifest itself the same in any two individuals. Rather, each individual must face the challenge of adaptation to capacities for returning to educational, vocational, recreational, social, and/or community life with a unique set of physical and psychological deficits.

The composite clients introduced earlier in this chapter embody just some of the many facets of premorbid, injury, and post-injury characteristics that influence the recovery of an individual. Recall any composite client. Each had premorbid characteristics of demographic background information, but also indicators of cultural or environmental heritage that affects even the manner in which the individual will react to injury and rehabilitation. Support networks ranged from a more normal family structure to tangled webs of relationships; each relationship bears an imprint upon the rehabilitation process. Personal information such as financial support or pending litigation bring multiple factors into rehabilitation consideration.

The brain, our center of "being-ness," is uniquely created and though weighing approximately three pounds, controls our every thought, action, and emotion. Although the general structure of the brain is alike from one brain to the next, there are no two identical responses to brain injuries. The individual having survived the trauma of brain injury is just beginning the uphill battle when medically stable. The reintegration into one's community requires successfully navigating many roadblocks from personal daily living skills, such as dressing and eating, to organizational and memory skills, to social skills. In order to reach the reintegration goal the individual must be an active participant in his own rehabilitation.

This engagement has often been labeled, "motivation to participate." Motivation, momentum, is that feeling one gets right before one fully understands a situation. This feeling, momentum, is created through the synergy generated among many qualities of four categories: one's perception of self, perception of recovery, vision, and interactions. Sustained momentum produces active engagement in rehabilitation activities, which, in turn, assists the individual in reaching the best quality of post-injury life possible.

In the final chapter, I discuss the results of this study in light of the relevant literature and offer recommendations for further research in this area.

CHAPTER 6

DISCUSSION

"At least we're fortunate, we can do stuff to forget."

-Milton, Windy Hill client

Introduction

The plight of individuals who have suffered traumatic brain injury (TBI) is difficult to capture in words. Metaphors, though powerful linguistic tools, likewise fall short in fully portraying the emotional, mental, physical, and spiritual pursuit of recovery experienced by the TBI community. Time stood still for me as a researcher, and as a TBI survivor, when Milton made the above comment. Yes, we, the traumatically brain injured, are fortunate. "We can do stuff to forget." The extent to which we classify ourselves, "fortunate" is dependent upon our definition of recovery, our ability to "do stuff." Through the constant comparative analysis procedures of grounded theory methods, I have been able to identify and unite factors relating to the motivation of individuals with TBI that enable them to "do stuff."

In the three studies reported in this dissertation without exception, the goal of every TBI participant has been to reconstruct their own lives to discover the "new me." Each survivor perceives and struggles to achieve some level of independence. These findings were consistent with the results of Nochi (1997) that he labeled "loss of self." To meet the challenges that lie ahead, the survivor of TBI must ultimately let go of his/her past "self" and begin again building on strengths that remain from his/her premorbid state thereby creating a new independence.

It is the sustained energy created by these processes of beginning again and creating that constitute at a global level the motivation to engage in rehabilitation. My investigation led to a primary insight not previously focused on in the existing literature on motivation, that a complex synergistic dynamic interplay of variables can either build on each other to create a momentum toward recovery, or can impede forward movement and grind recovery-enhancing actions to a halt.

The reciprocal relationship that exists between motivation and momentum is in itself one of the defining qualities of momentum, the central phenomenon. Momentum is a property of motivation, and as a property has an effect upon motivation. The motivational *triggers,* what causes the action, each contribute to the building of momentum. As the momentum gains in force, it catalyzes more motivational triggers and the process begins again. The critical value of understanding momentum is that all momentum is not necessarily good, or positive. In the case of the rehabilitation of individuals with traumatic brain injury, often behaviors are disruptive or inappropriate and the momentum gained in these negative traits can become as destructive on the one hand as constructive on the other. The value of momentum as a construct lies in its usefulness for behavioral direction. Because the inertia of one's actions appears to be created as momentum builds, either positively or negatively, it can be guided by monitoring the momentum characteristics. Recall the examples of Todd and Ellis (Figure 5.8, 5.9). The ultimate momentum in each example had survived and been built upon a series of events, not just one event. This compilation of a series of motivational events allowed an analysis for the direction of momentum at many steps along the way and opportunity to reverse negative forces. This compilation is afforded by the complexity and resilence of motivation. The continued growth of an individual in a rehabilitative program is similar to that of a young learner, that is, they profit from mistakes and gain momentum from each success. The engaged individual is one who is able to analyze his/her efforts which allows the individual to enjoy the optimal experience of flow in life (Csikszentmihalyi, 1990).

In the next section I begin by reviewing the findings of this study and the relationship of these findings to the current literature. I then move to implications for the field of rehabilitation and recommendations for further study.

Summary of Research Findings

When patients fail to comply with physician directives, when clients show little or no progress in rehabilitation programs, and when individuals in general show little attention to personal wellness concerns, the attribution is often made to the "unmotivated" individual (Jenny, 1983; Mikhail, 1981; Mullinax, 1995; Nobel & Hamilton, 1983; Pommier, 1992; Prochaska, 1994; Trostle, 1988; Ylvisaker & Gobble, 1987). While I agree that these reasons for poor behavior could be a result of the *unmotivated* individual, I propose that perhaps the label unmotivated masks the depth or breath of the real problem. As discussed in Chapter 2, the importance of motivation has long been recognized in the related fields of medicine. Largely due to the catastrophic nature of TBI, functional recovery following brain injury has certainly received attention by researchers who have acknowledged the importance of motivation in recovery (e.g. Ashley & Krych, 1995; Edelstein & Couture, eds, 1983; Prigatano, 1986). Clinicians have gradually eroded the myth that the central nervous system is a static, all-or-none unit. Potential has been expanded for functional recovery in the individual with TBI through the implementation of rehabilitation programs based on behavior theories and other learning theories (Berrol, in Prigatano, 1986, p. xvi). The debate continues on whether or not, and how much, the neurophysiology of TBI influences motivation in recovery. While such knowledge as a particular lesion diagnosis may be beneficial to the planning of rehabilitation initiation, the overlapping complexity of the cortical functions that direct everyday life should not be forgotten. Rather than an individual's motivation springing from one source or another, it appears to be, at least for the population represented in these data, the by-product of a vast number of combinations of one's daily perceptions.

This study was designed to address the following research question: What is the genesis and nature of the motivation experienced by individuals with traumatic brain injury in rehabilitation? The overarching finding is the theory of motivation that was generated from the data and is represented in the gyroscopic model. These data indicated that motivation catalyzes a synergy, which is generated from the relationships of innumerable personal characteristics of each individual. This synergy creates a reciprocal relationship to motivation that I labeled momentum. While the data yielded many rich insights into origins and relationships represented by the research question, I have selected three findings for exploration in this chapter: complexity, resilience, and the explication of the contextual category of perception of self. By complexity, I mean the multifarious, sophisticated, and compounded nature of the events that generate momentum. Resilience, then, represents the momentum-generating events that have qualities of flexibility, adaptability, and elasticity. The explication of the perception of self contextual category illustrates some of the unique features of the genesis of motivation.

I have selected these three areas for discussion because the examination of the complexity and resilience of momentum offers insight into the nature of motivation in this TBI population while the genesis of motivation is reflected in the explanation of perception of self. To probe the areas of complexity and resilience emphasizes the global nature of the findings. The scrutiny given to the contextual category perception of self focuses upon the practical workings of the model and offers a connection to the existing literature.

Finally, prior to the global discussion of the results, I offer a recap of the characteristics of the theory suggested by the data in this study. From the insights gained in working closely with 64 TBI clients in this study over a period of nine months, the outcome of motivation was *engagement* in rehabilitation programs. The data in this study suggested that engagement was achieved as a result of a synergy that was interactionally created by four contextual categories: (1) one's *perception of self, (2) perception of recovery, (3) vision,* and *(4) personal interactions.* This synergy was called *momentum,* the central phenomenon.

The interactional relationships of this study were metaphorically illustrated by a gyroscope, reflecting the momentum necessary to generate and maintain movement, or progress toward one's rehabilitation goal(s). The outcomes of momentum generate continued rehabilitation engagement that, in turn, enable the client to gain a new level of independence and to return to community life at the highest level possible.

Complexity of Momentum

A major finding of this study is that of the complexity of factors that influence and constitute motivation. Emerging from my data was a view of the momentum of motivation as not linear. Other models of motivation mostly presented in the educational literature, such as Schunk's motivated learning (1989); Eccles' achievement motivation (1983); or Harter's mastery motivation in children (1981), while thought provoking, do not capture the dimension of dynamism and the reciprocal influences of sub-components that were suggested by my data. The complexity of what encompasses motivation, represented in my choice of momentum for the core category, is due to the layered and interlocking feature of an individual's cognitive functions and circumstances across the dimension of time.

Perhaps at this point, a brief explanation of the reciprocal relationship between motivation at a global level and momentum at a systemic level would be helpful. As a concept, motivation is said to initiate behavior (Petri, 1991). A sustained behavior, particularly if successful, creates momentum. Momentum over time generates an increased volition, or movement to action. Because this relationship (motivation, momentum, and volition) is cyclical, it can be argued that momentum is the initiator for motivation that, in turn, generates volition.

293

The debate of where the cycle begins, however, is not the focus of this study, but rather it is an observation of the cyclical nature. The relationship of the phenomenon represented in these data indicate that the complex and deep-level characteristics of the subcategories are various forms of motivation, each of which can be a catalyst for generating momentum. The goal, then, is to sustain the momentum long enough to generate action in rehabilitative efforts, engagement.

Medical and rehabilitation caregivers, as well as members of the support network for an individual with TBI should be aware of the depth and complexity of the interworking parts that comprise motivation-generating momentum. In moving down the levels of the rotary disc of the gyroscope (Figure 5.2), one can obtain an understanding of each contextual category, with each category being illustrated on its own disc. Due to the complexity of the model, I did not illustrate levels beyond the general context. For example, Figure 6.1 illustrates the portion of Figure 5.2 showing the subcategories of the contextual category, Perception of Recovery. The structural decomposition of this same category is represented in Figure 6.2. To clarify the value of the structural decomposition to understanding the momentum of an individual's motivation, I have separated the three subcategories (stages of recovery, achievement, and gauntlets) and offer both a verbal and a graphic illustration of the decomposition process. Figures 6.3a and 6.3b are representative of the stages of recovery; Figures 6.4a and 6.4b show the decomposition of the subcategory of achievement; and finally, Figures 6.5a and 6.5b represent the analysis of the gauntlets.

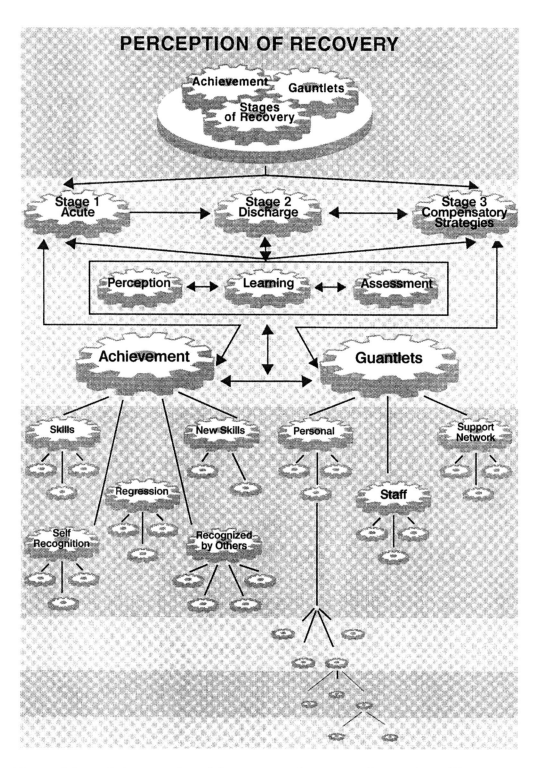

Figure 6.1.   Subcategories of the contextual category, Perception of Recovery

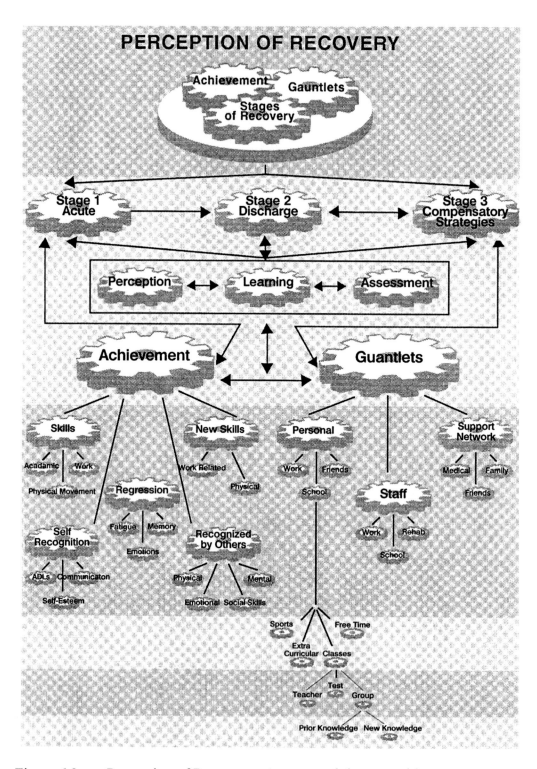

Figure 6.2.   Perception of Recovery: A structural decomposition

Stages of Recovery

Stage 1 Acute
* Hospital Staff
* Prognosis
* Diagnosis
* Visitors

Stage 2 Discharge
* Awareness of Time Restrictions
  * Physical
  * Social
  * Emotional
  * Mental
* Support Structure
  * Family
  * Friends
  * Medical
  * Rehab

Stage 3 Compensatory Strategies
* Time
* Community Involvement
  * Activities
  * Acceptance
  * Freedom
* Support Structure
  * Family
  * Friends
  * Medical
  * Rehab

Perception of Recovery
* Self
* Professional
* Family (support)

Learning Experiences
* Audio
* Visual
* Positive/ Negative

Assessment of Progress
* Self
* Professional
* Family

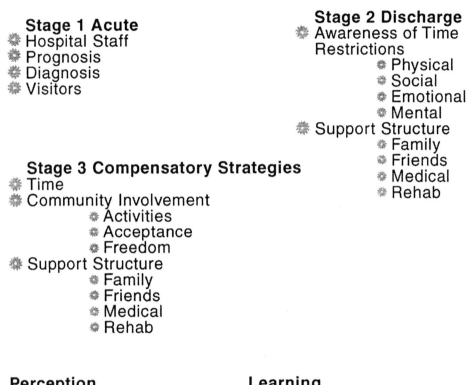

Figure 6.3a.   Stages of recovery: A verbal description

297

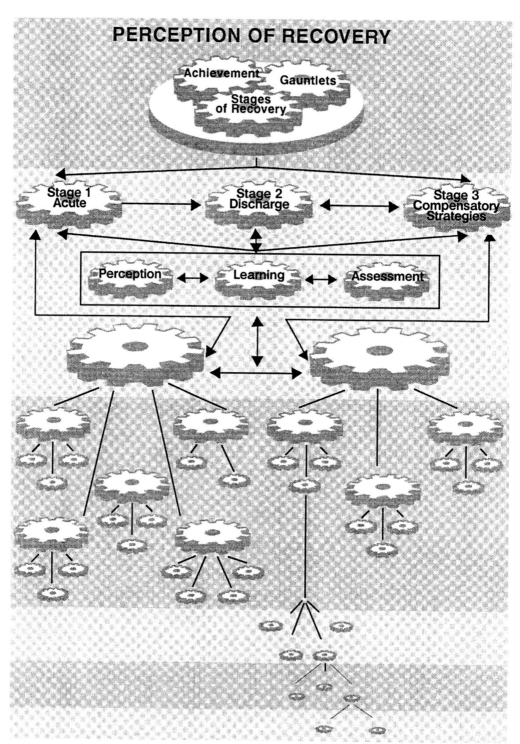

Figure 6.3b. Stages of recovery :
A graphic description

Achievement

Skills
- Physical Movement
    - Walking
    - Lifting
    - Sitting
- Work
    - Typing
    - Organizing
- Academic
    - Study
    - Reading
    - Computer

Self-Recognition
- ADLs
    - Brushing Teeth
    - Dressing
    - Personal Hygiene
- Communication
    - Phone
    - Personal
- Self- Esteem
    - High
    - Low

Regression
- Fatigue
- Memory
- Emotions
    - Anger
    - Depression
    - Temper

New Skills
- Work Related
    - Trade Skills
    - Organizational
- Physical
    - Compensatory Strategies
    - Regaining Abilities

Recognized By Others
- Physical
    - Movement
    - Compensation
- Mental
    - Memory
    - Conversation
- Emotional
    - Control
- Social Skills
    - Manners
    - Appropriate

Figure 6.4a.   Achievement: A verbal description

299

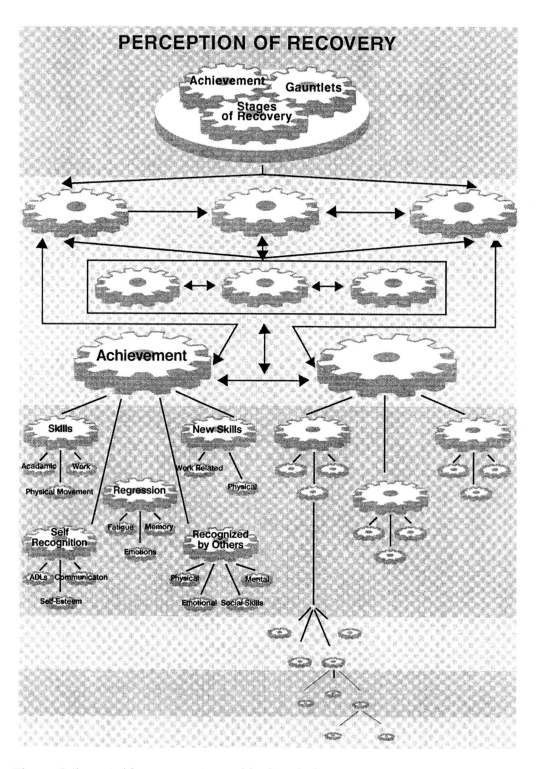

Figure 6.4b.   Achievement: A graphic description

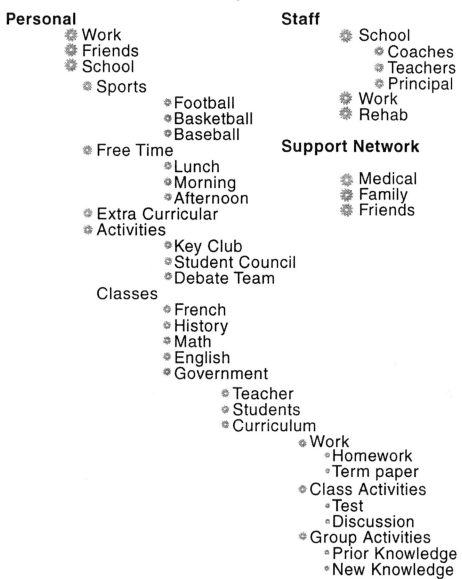

Gauntlets
✿ Perceived by Self
✿ Perceived by Others

Personal
✿ Work
✿ Friends
✿ School
  ✿ Sports
          ✿Football
          ✿Basketball
          ✿Baseball
  ✿ Free Time
          ✿Lunch
          ✿Morning
          ✿Afternoon
  ✿ Extra Curricular
  ✿ Activities
          ✿Key Club
          ✿Student Council
          ✿Debate Team
    Classes
          ✿French
          ✿History
          ✿Math
          ✿English
          ✿Government
              ✿Teacher
              ✿Students
              ✿Curriculum
                  ✿Work
                    ✿Homework
                    ✿Term paper
                  ✿Class Activities
                    ✿Test
                    ✿Discussion
                  ✿Group Activities
                    ✿Prior Knowledge
                    ✿New Knowledge

Staff
              ✿ School
                  ✿ Coaches
                  ✿ Teachers
                  ✿ Principal
              ✿ Work
              ✿ Rehab

Support Network

              ✿ Medical
              ✿ Family
              ✿ Friends

Figure 6.5a.   Gauntlets: A verbal description

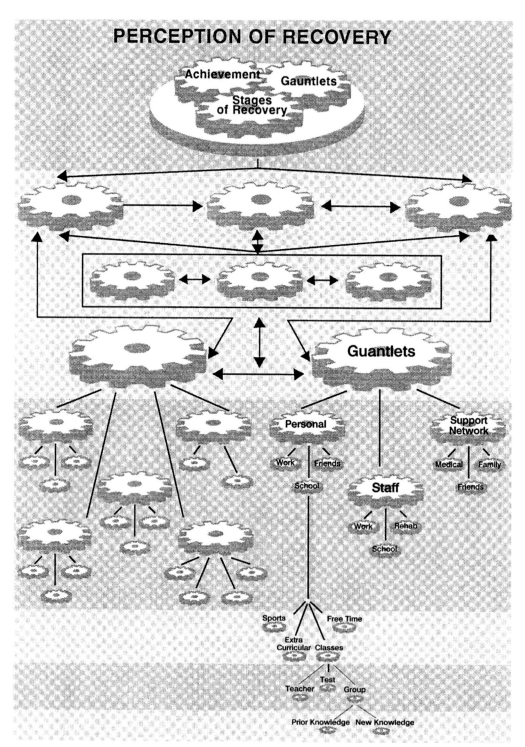

Figure 6.5b.   Gauntlets:
A graphic description

302

Note within the multiple layers that interact, that as one looks down the hierarchy the concepts become narrower, while looking upward, the concepts become broader. For example, note that the three stages of recovery all interact with the categories of current perception of recovery, learning experiences, and assessment of progress. In addition to each stage interacting with those subactivities, they also interact with the multiple layers of achievement and gauntlets. An individual in Stage 1 (acute) of recovery generally interacts with the subcategories in light of his/her acute status. However, the components of Stages 2 and 3 interact with each other at the same time as they are interacting with all the other subcategories. That is, an individual with TBI may drift between Stages 2 and 3 several times before gaining enough momentum to propel him/herself into the goal, community reentry. Looking closer at Figure 6.2, note that the subactivity of "personal" under gauntlets may have many subactivities itself, for example: acquaintances at work, friends, and schoolmates. Each of these subactivities will carry its own subactivities, such as school activities which may be divided into classes, free time, extracurricular, or sports and then divided again. For example, classes may be divided into teacher activity, test activity, and group activity. Learning in the group may be divided into prior knowledge and new knowledge. Herein lies the beauty of the complexity of the momentum of motivation. Let us survey this complexity through the experiences of Rod. (Figure 6.3)

Rod, one of my Tallangatta clients, has achieved a level of competence that allows him to be enrolled in the local high school mainstream classes. Let us place Rod in a group activity, seven levels removed from the contextual category of "Perception of Recovery." At the broad level of perception of recovery, it is difficult to pinpoint the source of motivation or demotivation in a particular activity other than to note Rod's comments or actions regarding the topic. Now Rod is in a senior government class and the group to which he has been assigned is reporting on the achievements of the current and the immediate past Presidents of the United States. The discussion progresses and all is well until one of the group asks Rod if the last President was a Democrat or Republican. Rod replies, "Heck, who was the last President?" because his memory cannot fill in that bit of information. Now, because Rod has a winsome personality illuminated with a quick wit and good looks, the girls in the group laugh and one young lady quickly answers, filling in, not only the President but also the party affiliation. Group activity continues and Rod actively participates. During the course of the remainder of the work session, Rod escapes several other basic questions through his humor. The group may be unaware of Rod 's sinking feeling of confidence resulting from his lack of knowledge on simple questions, his comparison of himself to his classmates, and his concern that he is not yet "recovering" as he had hoped. Rod's eroding self-confidence, then, becomes a demotivator at Level 7, which begins to slow down the positive rotation of a small "cog" in his "motivation gyroscope."

Now imagine that by the time Rod arrives at football practice, one of his coaches innocently yells out, "Hey, Rod, hope you've got those new plays in the memory bank." Now a larger "cog" at Level 5 is slowing its positive rotation, for Rod's confidence in his memory erodes even more as he interprets the coach's joking as serious and fears he may not remember the new plays. Rod has no way of knowing that the coach had said the exact same thing to every team member as he took to the practice field. Earlier in the day, Rod was feeling on top of the world in Stage 3, Level 1, and a very positive momentum was building. Now, at day's end, through a series of smaller, seemingly insignificant events, Rod has dropped back to Stage 2 in his inner drive, for he has decided that his learning strategies, Level 2, are poor and he cannot compete with normal classmates. At the close of the day, the support network around Rod inquires why he looks so sad, or why he is moping about. Rod replies, "Ah, nothing, I just can't remember the new football plays." Members of his support network, then, can respond to this statement, in one of many ways that at this time limit his momentum. "Well, you just have to try harder," or "Sure, just work on your memory, it will happen," or "Don't worry, all the guys have problems with new plays," or "If you're motivated enough, you'll do it, hang in there." By this time Rod, after hours of frustration, finds himself losing that momentum without knowing exactly why. The negative torque of his motivational gyroscope has slowed enough cogs, small to large, that it is impeding his progress. After a time, then, we recognize Rod as an unmotivated client because "he just does not see himself getting better. He must see it first." Therefore, from the innocent laughter of classmates responding to his antics to cover his inadequate memory to a coach kidding with him, to a support member encouraging him to "hang in there," Rod has lost momentum. While the example is perhaps oversimplified, it represents the model I have presented, and is, in fact, taken directly from my observational notes with only the sport being changed to protect Rod's privacy.

A scenario as above may seem improbable in the course of daily living; however, I remember a similar happening early in my return to academic life

305

when my classmates all wanted to go see the movie *Nixon*. When I asked what it was about, they all laughed and replied, "The President, crazy." I laughed, and I, too, being the group clown, escaped any further embarrassment, but to myself, thought "the President of what?" I had no recollection of the years of President Nixon. A barometer for my recovery, the internal comparison of self to others, gnawed at me until I gracefully declined attending the movie. The challenge for the individual with TBI is that in the midst of the situation, it is often impossible to realize that an event as just described is simply a piece of missing memory rather than a learning deficit or indication of lack of progress.

Consider again the story of Rod. Let us suppose now that the support network member offered a different reply to Rod's declaration of his memory problem with the football plays. Instead of offering any number of general motivational "throwaway lines," imagine that the worker had stopped for just a minute to inquire about the problem and, in the course of the conversation, discovered the events of the day. The scenario might have turned out differently. Rod could have been guided to a new compensatory strategy for his weak memory, using strategies for relearning rather than retreating. The support member must become a "detective on duty" at all times when assisting a TBI individual to regain independence. I do not intend to leave the impression that this dissection is necessary, or possible, in every situation. Rather I am saying that the complexity of momentum allows for it to be redirected if support workers are aware of the depth of the motivational resources of an individual. In the illustrative case of Rod, it took an entire day to grind his momentum gyroscope to a halt. At any point during that time, it could have been regenerated rather easily.

I have chosen to call the events that build an individual's momentum, his/her motivation quotient. This quotient, or ratio of positive events to negative events, should be monitored by those in supportive roles with individuals recovering from TBI. Individuals having survived TBI usually cannot analyze elements that tend to discourage them, especially in their perceptions of self or their perceptions of recovery.

Systemic Resilience of Momentum

The complexity of the momentum of motivation is built upon the foundations of its systemic resilience. Graphically each of the four contextual categories has been illustrated as a group of cogs interlocking with other cogs to generate the momentum of the gyroscope. However, the unique element of each interlocking cog is that the TBI survivor has "an ability to recover from or adjust easily to misfortune or change" (Merriam-Webster, 1993, p. 996) in order to link with one of the other cogs. Translated to the life of an individual with TBI, this means that the motivators, as well as the demotivators, can be shaped in many different ways. Systemic resilience illustrates the flexibility of momentum in the face of obstacles. In selecting the term resilience to describe this phenomenon of motivation, I am not using the term in the review of the literature published by the Basic Behavioral Science Task Force for the National Advisory Mental Health Council (1996).

The nature of resilience can be seen in all aspects of the model. I will explore it as it was expressed in the contextual category of Vision. This category suggested three components: spiritual vision, achievement vision (goals), and vision of hope and humor. For illustrative purposes, the component of achievement vision (goals) is discussed because the data offered so many rich examples of what I have labeled resilience.

The differences in goal expectations were an interesting discovery in these data as they relate to resilience. Goal theory has provided a framework for the study of motivation in educational research. The goal patterns studied by Meece and Holt (1993) were easily recognizable in this population. In a study of 257 fifth and sixth grade students, Meece and Holt (1993) identified three different goal patterns exhibited by the students: task-mastery, ego-social, and work-avoidant. Task mastery goals "represent a desire to learn something new, master a task, or improve one's competence" (p. 582). Ego-social goals represent "a desire to demonstrate high ability or to please the teacher" (p. 582). Those with work-avoidance goals "seek to complete their [students'] work with a minimum of effort" (p. 582). While individuals with TBI can engage in each of the three goal patterns in varying stages of their rehabilitation program all at the same time, a common indicator of progress, no matter which goal pattern they follow, is their response to the misfortune of not reaching the goal or of having the goal redirected. This response I have labeled resilience. The behavior modification efforts experienced in training Joe to tidy his room represent resilience through all three patterns.

Joe, a client from Windy Hill, was 15 years post-injury and had overcome many recovery obstacles. Joe was a great example of someone who was happier with life now than pre-accident because of a checkered premorbid history with the negative events far outweighing the positive events in his life. Joe had overcome strife in his unhappy family relationships, his self-efficacy had blossomed, and he had learned a work ethic that any employer would appreciate. However, one area of Joe's life remained a deep problem. He had tremendous difficulty in keeping his room tidy. His room was always in a state of disarray. The unmade bed was the backdrop for the apple cores, wadded up bits of paper, dirty clothes, toiletry supplies, untold books, and "stuff." These items were like a ribbon encircling the room and winding its way to the bathroom where another equally messy room began. I do not refer to this mess as one would refer to typical untidiness. Perhaps the word "shambles" should be used as the adjective of choice. Joe was reminded time and again to clean his room. Reminders failed, though Joe was cheerful each time he was reminded and replied, "Yep, OK." In the initial stages, staff felt that perhaps Joe was avoiding the work of cleaning his room with his cheerful response to direction. Seeing reminders did not work, staff soon turned to docking his token pay for each day he left his room unkempt. Again, the method failed. While Joe lost money regularly on his room, he was making a great deal of token money because other aspects of his program earned him rewards, so he did not miss the token deduction very much. However, the regular reminding by the staff and deduction of money began to irritate him. After watching Joe carefully in his room-cleaning habits, it became obvious that he really was anxious to please the staff, thus his cheerful attitude initially when he was reminded. Sensing the problem then was rooted deeper than just "forgetfulness," the staff learned that Joe actually did not know how to clean his room. Joe often thought his room was tidy for he had moved a few things around and the mounds and stacks were gone; therefore the room must be clean. Fortunately, Joe was resilient and cheerfully tried each new attempt to assist his memory, not realizing the real problem was not memory alone but skills that needed to be relearned.

Finally, the idea surfaced to create a checklist for Joe listing the steps with which to clean his room properly. A chart, HOUSEKEEPING, was made and laminated, that allowed Joe the opportunity to make notes on this chart. A Vis-a-Vis™ pen was attached to the chart for ease of making notes. The chart had three categories: Chore, Steps, Done. Each cleaning chore had its own entry on the chart and a notation was made listing the requirements for proper cleaning in the "steps" space. For example, the category "shelves" listed "books neatly stacked, no loose papers, CD's stacked, no clothes." Then the section, "done" was available for Joe to check to indicate he had accomplished that task. Staff then checked the chart at some time during the day while Joe was at work and if Joe had a clean room, with chart completed, then he received bonus money at the end of the day. After Joe had successfully remembered the "steps" in any "chore" category for a period of weeks, the "steps" section of the chart was blocked leaving just the reminder of the chore to be completed. Joe had control over his life for he knew if he did not complete the checklist prior to leaving for work, there would be no reward at day's end. Over a period of time, Joe repeated the task enough that it became habit and eventually, the chart was discarded. (This is not to imply, however, that the room was always tidy!).

The resilience of momentum is illustrated in Joe's case by the number of solutions attempted before finding the best solution to the dilemma of performing and mastering housekeeping chores. In this case, the pliable nature of Joe's motivation actually allowed the momentum to swing both positively and negatively until the right type of assistance was discovered. Motivation is not necessarily a particular type such as intrinsic or extrinsic, but often a combination of several types all bending and blending together. The resilience of momentum allows an individual to achieve success even in light of many unsuccessful attempts.

Consider again the value of the "zone of proximal development" (Vygotsky, 1978) discussed in Chapter 2, now in relation to resilience. When an individual accepts the challenge to develop a new competency, not just repeat the old ones, and has a knowledgeable mentor in proximity, he/she has entered the "zone of proximal development" according to Vygotsky. According to Vygotsky, the zone of proximal development is "[the] distance between the actual developmental level as determined by independent problem solving and the level of potential development as determined through problem solving under adult guidance or in collaboration with capable peers" (1978, p. 86). From this Vygotskian concept was born the idea of "scaffolding," that is gradual withdrawal of control or supervision of the scaffolder as the mastery level of the scaffoldee increases (Meyer, 1993). This tool is particularly helpful with the individual suffering from TBI for suddenly he/she has been placed in a learner's role for skills long ago mastered. The benefits of scaffolding are that in addition to being pliable, information or help can be given just at the time it is needed. In this manner, the recovering client with TBI is not overwhelmed with information, thereby reaching overload and quitting, which would be counterproductive to building motivation momentum. Scaffolding allows for the motivational factors to be monitored and their resilient nature to be harnessed for gaining momentum.

By using the technique of scaffolding, the chances increase for keeping the recovering TBI individual within the *flow* of his/her life. Flow occurs for any individual when they "are so involved in an activity that nothing else seems to matter…" (Csikszentmihalyi, 1990, p. 4). Any engaging event can assist in maintaining the flow experience. The longer the rehabilitative efforts of an individual continue to provide the optimal experiences in reconstructing his/her life, the longer the rehabilitation progress can be sustained. Reconstructing one's life is based upon regaining old knowledge and gaining new knowledge. According to Meyer (1993), "knowledge is a constructive process for giving personal meaning to experience; …our interactions within a particular context influence our construction of knowledge; and…neither knowledge nor context remains stable, but co-evolve as a natural part of human interaction and development" (p. 41-42). Therefore, according to the processes proposed by Meyer (1993), scaffolding does include negotiation of meaning and the transfer of responsibility for learning to the learner. Scaffolding the learning processes for the individual with TBI is a socio-constructive concept for it is collaborative and provides optimal experiences for client engagement and choice while being non-evaluative. To be resilient is to be flexible, adaptable in circumstances. Scaffolding allows the mentor to monitor the mentee and use the flexibility and adaptability of the motivational factors present to guide the learning process. The essence of this co-evolving knowledge is key in the strength of the resilience of momentum.

Explication of Perception of Self

This study identified five components of one's perception of self: (1) ability, (2) value, (3) perception of premorbid self, (4) acceptance of self as injured, and (5) fear. There are untold hundreds of studies on one's identity of self in the annals of psychology journals. The mystery of the self and society's pursuit of the solution to that mystery sustains many researchers, psychologists, and psychiatrists in business. The strongest link in the literature to this study was the 1997 study of Nochi, *Loss of Self: A Narrative Study on People with Traumatic Brain Injuries*. Nochi worked with and interviewed 10 TBI survivors. Qualitative analysis of his data revealed four interrelated categories of loss of self: (1) loss of single self-history, (2) opaque self, (3) devalued self, and (4) labeled self. Nochi posited that the individual's self-history could follow either of two contradictory schools of thought: either it is continuous despite TBI, or it is discontinuous because of TBI. In defining the opaque self of TBI survivors, Nochi suggested that the individual with TBI has lost clear self-knowledge and is uncertain of his/her role in society both in the present and the future. For Nochi's third category, the devalued self, TBI survivors tend to compare themselves with pre-injury selves in terms of interpersonal relations, job capacities, etc., and feel that their present selves are valueless. Nochi's fourth category, the labeled self, indicates that an individual with TBI may sense that society presses upon them negative labels that contradict their own self-images.

In my study, I found similar struggles. For example, the acceptance of self as "injured" (labeled self) was shown in the following: "I'm not a patient, I'm not

313

a client, I'm a person. So, I've had an injury but I'm like everyone else. I have the same needs, wants, and desires. Why do I get treated like a prisoner and everyone is telling me what to do? I can run my own life and right now, my goal is to get my degree" (Wally). In my study, one's perception of self had five dimensions, similar categories to those of Nochi for four, and a fifth category, "fear" (of growth and recovery), was added. As Darrell once expressed, "we can come up with ideas. Some of us are scared, worn out because we got this group [and we keep each other scared]. Everybody's afraid they'll just walk out and then be alone."

In addition to the research of Nochi, another guiding force for the definition of this category was the literature on self-efficacy. According to Bandura, self-efficacy is "a judgment of one's capability to accomplish a certain level of performance" (1998). For the individual with TBI, this personal "judgment of one's capability" is directly linked to his/her perception of his/her recovery at any given time. When one's self-efficacy is higher, so is the synergistic nature of the individual's activities and efforts. The danger of loss of momentum for the individual with TBI is readily apparent in light of the issue of self-efficacy.

Recall the self-determination theory of Deci and Ryan (1991), the individual having a choice, or at least feeling that he/she has a choice is more likely to have a motivated behavior as opposed to a controlled, intentional behavior often called compliance. It is important to guide the rehabilitation of an individual with TBI; however, it is equally important that the individual has a sense of self-control in his/her program.

In a lighthearted moment, this issue of the client feeling that he is in control of his life was highlighted with Stan. Stan had drawn the ire of a female staff member for playfully "pinching her bottom." Certainly this behavior is not appropriate, and Stan was reprimanded and lost privileges for a period of time. Because Stan and I have worked together closely over months, I asked him about the incident days later. I inquired to see if he remembered it at all and if so, what explanation he would give. In his witty manner, he flashed his devilish grin, assured me he would never do that to me and then offered, "Yep, I remember. It felt good. She had made me mad by telling me I was unrealistic in my dreams…(pause, obviously thinking) I know it was wrong, but for that one moment, I was in charge! When I'm good, I'm really good, when I'm bad, I'm really bad! I'll make it because I can see me making it in the future." The twinkle in his eye melted any additional reprimand I had planned. I chuckled to myself knowing he was right; I could remember feeling good to be in control in rehabilitation situations, even if it meant rebelling at times.

Recall the kaleidoscope in Chapter 5; it had been broken and no longer yielded geometrically balanced and beautiful designs in a prism of colors; instead it was like arcs that would no longer intersect but came ever so close. The bits and pieces of a TBIer's broken kaleidoscope are the very genesis of his/her motivation. The challenge is to find a piece that one can build upon and, though a painfully slow process one piece at a time, the individual with traumatic brain injury can rebuild his/her kaleidoscope, not necessarily to yield the original beautiful designs, but workable, unique designs nonetheless.

Limitations of Study

The three potential limitations for this study are environmental, longitudinal, and personal.

ENVIRONMENTAL

This study was conducted at a rehabilitation facility that specializes in brain injury rehabilitation. The philosophy of this rehabilitation facility is based on the token economy system, in which each client begins earning from the first day he/she arrives. The rehabilitation environment is one of a therapeutic nature. Clients accepted into this program must meet the following criteria:

- Eighteen years of age or older (ages 16 and 17 evaluated for appropriateness)
- Medically stable
- Prognosis to ambulate with assistance
- Not dangerous to oneself and/or others
- Continent of bowel and bladder for the majority of the time
- Funding secured

The selectivity and the nature of the program itself should be considered in the transfer of any interpretation from this study. The motivational factors for clients not fortunate enough to meet the admission criteria and/or have access to a therapeutic environment could vary from those reported by these individuals. I hasten to say, however, that for the participants in both my Preliminary Studies, many of whom never had any formal rehabilitation beyond Stage 1 (acute) recovery, the motivational factors named in this study are consistent with the feelings reported in the earlier studies. The rehabilitation network's structure of daily activities was a major factor in the success of these individuals. A change in rehabilitation facility structure or a lack of formal rehabilitation structure of any kind could, and perhaps would, influence the factors of motivation.

LONGITUDINAL

While the three studies reported in this dissertation span 17 months, and the primary study occurred during 9 of those 17 months, the nature of long-term recovery from a traumatic brain injury is much longer than 9 months. The probable limitations from such a relatively short observation were, in part, countered by the fact that the clients with whom I worked were all more than one-year post-injury. Because recovery from traumatic brain injury is such a long process, the real characteristics of one's motivational tendencies will not show up in the first 12-18 months post-injury. During these first months the individual is wrestling with the long-term nature of his/her disability and the motivational tendencies are not necessarily stabilized. Nonetheless, a longitudinal study over years of an individual's recovery experiences would certainly lend more strength to the interpretations.

PERSONAL

Finally, while I strongly believe that the emic knowledge from my personal experience over the past 13 years as a traumatic brain injury survivor was a strength of this study, I must recognize that it is possible that my interpretations of the participants' perceptions were unduly colored by my own experiences. To test the durability of my findings, perhaps a non-TBI individual could examine the theoretical model in a similar setting. According to Strauss and Corbin (1990), reproducibility of findings can be attempted in this manner: "[g]iven the same theoretical perspective of the original researcher and following the same general rules for data gathering and analysis, plus a similar set of conditions, another investigator should be able to come up with the same theoretical explanation about the given phenomenon" (p. 251).

Implications for Field of Rehabilitation

Two of the most frequently asked questions that I fielded related to long-term rehabilitation were (1) "what motivated you all those years in rehab?" and (2) "how can I motivate (name of patient, friend, or relative) who is now in a long-term rehabilitation situation?" My answer to the first question is simple: "God." With the model that has emerged from these data, I can now answer the second question without waffling among a multitude of ideas with no explicit support from which to choose. While this study focused on the motivational factors that would help someone recover from traumatic brain injury, I believe it offers three implications for the field of rehabilitation in general. These implications are: (1) the need for scaffolding momentum in long-term rehabilitation; (2) motivational awareness for one-on-one situations; and (3) the challenge to teach staff and client support members with hands-on ideas for motivating clients.

The categories and concepts presented in this study are not the only properties of motivational factors, but rather a starting point for the journey of uncovering the keys to motivating individuals suffering from traumatic brain injury as well as other long-term rehabilitative disabilities or illnesses. If rehabilitation specialists and support network members limit themselves to this model, they may miss some critical motivator for their client/family member/friend dealing with the frustrations of TBI rehabilitation. The categories and concepts presented in this study should serve as landmarks—directional points on a map sharpening the awareness of each TBI survivor. Just as there are no two brain injuries that are identical, there will be no two sets of motivational factors that are identical, but rather they will share the same landmarks or points on the map of recovery.

Unfortunately, in the field of health care often we tend to refer to an individual by his/her physical ailment(s): "the gun shot wound in trauma 4," "the gall bladder in 14," "the head lac [laceration] in 2." Each time one is addressed in this manner, whether in his/her presence or not, the unique characteristics of the individual, the very fibers of his/her being that make him/her an individual are overlooked. The momentum for motivation begins at the basic level of individual characteristics.

Consider the case of Peggy, three years post-injury. Peggy had made steady progress in her studies toward her GED (General Education Diploma) certification, her weight gain had stopped and she was beginning to experience success in her weight loss program, she had begun to feel valued as a person again after struggling through some tough times with her family network. Her months of rehabilitation efforts were beginning to be easily seen in her appearance, her speech, and her memory. For Peggy, life was beginning to be exciting again. I had the opportunity to work with Peggy on a number of occasions and often listened to her recount the obstacles she had overcome and those she yet had to conquer. One day we were at the washateria with the group and while the dryers were spinning several clients had gathered around and we were all enjoying general chit chat, nothing in particular. Peggy bent over and picked up a pad of POST IT NOTES ™ to tag a dryer with her name (all dryers were labeled with client names to assist staff in checking laundry with clients since clothes were laundered in a public washateria). Peggy began to quickly jot down her name in order to be able to rejoin the conversation and accidentally wrote on the side with the sticky strip used for posting the note to a surface. A staff member happened by at that point and noticed that Peggy had written on the wrong side of the POST IT NOTE™, and in an attempt to be humorous I'm sure, said, "Peggy, Peggy, Peggy, stupid, stupid, stupid, that is the wrong side of the note. Here use this side." At this point the staff member took the pad from Peggy and turned it over and handed it back to her. Peggy sat stunned, mouth open and staring at the staff member. Then she exclaimed, "What do you think I am? I'm not stupid, stupid, stupid" and began to fight back the tears. By this time the staff member had vanished from the general area of conversation and moved across the washateria to assist another client. The clients in our circle of conversation likewise jumped in and began to exclaim how unfair it had been to call Peggy stupid. For the remainder of the morning at the washateria, I spent time attempting to calm Peggy down and avoid any further crisis. One of Peggy's first comments was, "I am not stupid. I'm human and I'm worth something, aren't I?" Unfortunately, Peggy's immediate anger did not wash the hurt or negative imprint away from her mind. For the next several weeks, each time Peggy and I would be partnered, Peggy would perseverate upon the incident and as the days wore on she began to drift back into the meek Peggy of earlier days with little confidence and regular exclamations of the fact that "I'm not happy with my life…it's so pitiful…people who used to love me are gone…I know my surroundings and it is no family, no money, no home, no love…do you think I'm stupid, stupid, stupid?" In Peggy's motivational gyroscope, the self-efficacy cog had reversed its forward momentum and the negative torque was beginning to slow down not only that cog, but others that were related to it along the way. From that one thoughtless comment, Peggy had been set back several weeks in her progress due to circumstances she could not control as a TBI survivor, the feeling of value of self. Surely the staff member had only intended to guide Peggy with the POST IT NOTE™ episode; however, the interpretation Peggy experienced left her feeling she was not in control of her own life. Important to the self-esteem of an individual with TBI is the feeling that he/she is in control of his/her life.

In addition to the issue of the individual with TBI feeling a sense of the value of self, the issue of communication is important. Discussions of communication relationships in health care settings such as Emanuel and Emanuel (1992) or Northouse and Northouse (1992) allude to but never really define one of the key elements of communications. In light of these data, one of the keys to the success of rehabilitation efforts is that of the illocutionary and perlocutionary effectiveness of communications between the individual with TBI and his/her supportive team. Borrowing from the speech-act theory (Steinmann, Jr., 1982) illocutionary effectiveness is to have what you meant to say be understood. Perlocutionary effectiveness, on the other hand, means that the words move the listener to fulfill the intent of the utterance. The goal, then, for the rehabilitation worker is to say things that are not only understood (illocutionary effectiveness) but that actually move the patient to engage in action (perlocutionary effectiveness). During these months of data gathering, I witnessed two forms of ineffective illocutionary/perlocutionary speech that affected the momentum outcome for the individual.

The most common of ineffective effects was that of illocutionary speech; the individual simply did not understand the information being given to him/her. The complex relationship of the perlocutionary speech being ineffective surfaced in two ways. First, the word choice perhaps did not connect with the client in order to move him/her to action. For example, a staff member may say, "Grace, time to take your meds." To Grace, that did not translate, "go take my meds, now." While illocutionary effectiveness (understanding) was present in that example, the staff member rethinking his/her choice of words could alter the lack of perlocutionary effectiveness (action) easily enough. The other form of ineffective communication I observed between illocution and perlocution is more complex in its limitations to the growth of momentum.

Many clients, especially at the Tallangatta program, could clearly understand what was being said but just did not care to follow through for some reason or another. This "some reason or another" is the heart of the complexity of the multidimensional model that was generated from these data. The lack of motivation in many cases did not spring from perlocutionary ineffectiveness, but rather from some momentum trigger at say level 6 or 7 of an individual's life. This observation led me to notice that often the lack of momentum can be due to the differentiation between ability and effort.

Noting the work of Weiner (1994), this distinction can be illustrated by "the differentiation between characterological [what one is like] and behavioral [what one has done] blame…" (p.163). According to Weiner, ability and effort "differ in the causal property of controllability" (1994, p. 165). "ability…is not controllable by the individual—one cannot willfully become able or volitionally change one's ability. Effort, on the other hand, is a controllable cause of failure" (1994, p. 165). At times I noticed that interactions were labeled, "ineffective" and the client, "unmotivated," when the real problem was that the interpretation of the client to his/her ability was not in tune with that of the staff member, thereby making the client feel out of control of his/her own life and spurring the non-active response to communication. Herein is the value of scaffolding the individual along the rehabilitation pathway. If the individual is being scaffolded, then his/her abilities can be matched to his efforts and vice versa. This positive match, then, creates flow for the individual since he/she can become totally engaged in his/her activity.

Recommendations for Further Research

A theory of practice cannot become a tool for practice until it has passed formative and summative evaluation and revisions. Without testing, a theory remains just sets of data bound together by interpretation and speculation of what might work. I recommend three primary areas of focus for further research in this area: (1) confirming and/or expanding the contextual categories suggested by these data, (2) developing specific techniques for scaffolding motivation, and (3) exploring its application to other long-term rehabilitation situations. Therefore, even as the gyroscopic theory was emerging from my data sets, I began to test the concepts and seek some formative evaluations for myself in each of these categories.

CONFIRMING AND/OR EXPANDING THE CONTEXTUAL CATEGORIES

I selected three clients, Darrell, Todd, and Stan, for this first mini-test. The project was to involve a collaboration on the rebuilding of the Bonsai program at the network-owned nursery. These clients were selected for a variety of reasons. Darrell has been a nursery employee for over five years and was quite knowledgeable in the art of Bonsai; in fact, he was the nursery Bonsai manager. Neither Todd nor Stan had nursery experience prior to this project. They were selected primarily to see if such an experience could boost their self-perception through a feeling of achievement and value with a job outside of their token jobs at Windy Hill, their residential facility. Darrell was selected not only because he was the Bonsai manager, but also because of the need to sharpen his interpersonal skills and his ability to set and maintain commitment to personal goals.

The project commenced in January and is still in progress even as this dissertation is reaching its completion. I have maintained records on the progress of the trio, and it has been interesting to note that in the beginning stages all three were anxious to be involved simply for the excitement of a new challenge and the opportunity, and especially for the two Windy Hill clients, to be involved with me personally. The personal bond that had formed among the three of us was quite strong, but is expressed in different ways. I was interested to see if the personal bond that I shared with each of these young men could be shifted to each other and then to the project itself. In rehabilitation efforts it is important for the individual to ultimately want to be engaged for himself/herself, not to please a staff member.

I worked with Darrell approximately one month prior to the arrival of his two "workers." During this month, Darrell and I discussed his business plan for rebuilding the Bonsai business at the nursery, how to be a "boss" and a "friend," how to be a good mentor, how to use the fax machine (Darrell faxes me a daily update of the business progress), and how to keep focused: "If it is to be, it is up to me." Darrell and I spent time transplanting many young Bonsai. When we first began to involve the other two young men, I would sit with Darrell in his daily "instructional" sessions with Todd and Stan and then oversee the work of Todd and Stan. As time passed, Darrell learned and began to complete a "work report" for each of his assignees, and my direct involvement gradually declined.

It was fascinating to watch the momentum grow over the weeks and now months of this project. The clients instinctively encouraged each other at various levels of the grounded theory model I was testing and held in my head. For example, upon a day, Todd transplanted one Bonsai all by himself. Stan asked Darrell if he could try it and to my surprise Darrell replied, "Sure, can you remember the steps if I teach you?" Stan assured him he could remember. Darrell and Stan spent the afternoon transplanting with Stan repeating the various steps to him periodically. Darrell complimented him on his memory, thereby boosting his perception of self in the subcategory of achievement. The startling revelation to me, however, was the compliment from Todd to Stan. Rather than compliment him on his memory improvement, which was by far the most obvious daily improvement, Todd complimented Stan on his use of his weak-side hand. (Stan suffers from a partial hemiparesis and struggles to use one side of his body and to control muscular tremors.) Todd reached down several levels in the contextual category of definition of recovery, through Stage 2 (past learning experiences), and seized the opportunity to compliment Stan on a deep personal concern. The smile on Stan's face sent chills down my back, and the momentum gained would have been visible frame by frame had I been videotaping this session.

As time passed in this project, the young men all bonded to each other as they worked together, and moved away from just a connection with me. Finally, all three young men are becoming enthused about rebuilding this area of the business; this challenge is providing moments of optimal experience during work hours. While a complete discussion of this project is the subject for later analysis, I was pleasantly surprised to see the multidimensional model working so well.

DEVELOPING SPECIFIC TECHNIQUES FOR SCAFFOLDING MOTIVATION

My other mini-test was to create a situation in which motivation could be scaffolded. I wanted to see if a situation could be created in which an optimal experience would make any difference in motivation. I selected Stan as my Epworth client for this test. Stan was a university student prior to his accident. He remains highly intelligent and has a vocabulary that puts mine to shame. His major deficit, outside the physical gait difficulties, is his short-term memory. On occasion, throughout the months that I worked with Stan, I noticed that if something was important to him and he felt in charge, he strove to remember that particular item or task.

Therefore, I decided to link him with a young fifth grade boy, Jack, who had experienced acquired brain injury (congenital) and subsequent surgery. I selected a younger male with brain injury in order for Stan to feel his role as the mentor and not as competitor, in that Jack likewise had experienced injury. Jack also experiences some hemiparesis resulting from his surgery; therefore he and Stan had that in common. I instructed Stan that he was to mentor Jack on his schoolwork. I instructed Jack that he was to encourage Stan with his short-term memory. Again, this project is ongoing, but the insights gained in the short period of monitoring the progress of both of these young men has been exceptional.

I took Jack with me to work one day and this gave Jack and Stan time to get to know each other. Stan did like Jack and felt it important "to help him at school, since I'm still smart." Jack, though by his own admission a bit scared of Stan at first, felt important because as "only a fifth grader, I'm a researcher helping someone else with brain injury." The two planned Jack's forthcoming speech assignment and divided up the "responsibilities" for its completion. The project began routinely with Stan receiving cueing from staffers to remember to fax Jack to offer suggestions, and Jack eagerly awaiting reply from Stan. By my design, this project had an intriguing relationship built in. I was interested on the one hand to see if Stan's interest in Jack could spur his memory and if, on the other hand, the attention from Stan and the need to rise to a challenge greater than any he'd experienced before (a fifth grader mentoring a grown man) could propel Jack into the optimal experience described by Csikszentmihalyi (1990).

The data that are being gathered on this project exceed my expectations. After the first week of "cued" faxes from Stan and the replies from Jack, things appeared to fall apart. Jack stopped receiving faxes, he became a bit disappointed, then seemed to forget the project with Stan as his own speech deadline (presentation at school) was coming up quickly. Jack and I worked diligently at school on two occasions and prepared for his speech. During our work time, Jack questioned why Stan had not continued to fax and wondered if something could be wrong. Jack was curious to know if there was anything that he could do to change Stan faster. The plan that Stan and Jack had organized on their first visit called for some sophisticated visuals for a fifth grader! Therefore, I became quite involved in the preparation process to assist in finalizing the "plan." In the process of working, Jack became so involved with the new ways to make visuals for his speech he completely forgot his struggles with using his left side and began using his left arm a great deal more. Albeit still awkward, his left arm did not slow him down as I'd noticed in previous work sessions.

Upon returning to work the next week, I discovered to my horror that Stan had, in fact, remembered to write Jack daily regarding their project and that the staff had failed to send the faxes for him (as a client, he was not allowed to use the fax machine). Stan was hurting, feeling separated from his new mentee, and Jack was disappointed, for he felt he had failed. I spent time at the Windy Hill program straightening out the staff understanding and spent time discussing the problems with Jack and brainstorming possible solutions with him. I also enlisted the aid of Jack's parents to assist me in monitoring the arrival of any faxes so I could be informed immediately if a breakdown (other than Stan forgetting) occurred. When the problem was finally resolved, Stan was rejuvenated in his efforts to remember to fax Jack. As this dissertation concludes, these two are working on yet another project. This one is about brain injury. In addition to their connection on Jack's schoolwork, the two are sharing sporting, camping, movie, and guy-type stories by faxes. They hope to plan an outing to go to a movie together. The lessons to be gained in this project, I believe, are specific ways in which to scaffold the learning process for individuals with traumatic brain injury.

Conclusion

This is not the end but rather only the beginning. This dissertation has presented a new view of the dynamic nature of motivation. I received varied answers from clients as I would member check, share findings with them and solicit their input on results. While sharing with Stan some of the results of this study, I asked him what advice he would offer to individuals given the opportunity and the challenge to assist someone with TBI. He could not remember the exact words I had taught him when we were talking about his role in working with Jack, but he remembered the gist of it and said, "I'd tell them the walking thingy you told me." The "walking thingy," I believe summarizes the plea for all survivors of traumatic brain injury as they battle reconstructing self and re-entering community life:

> Don't walk in front of me, I may not follow,
> Don't walk behind me, I cannot lead,
> Just walk beside me and be my friend.

> —Unknown

APPENDICES

APPENDIX A

FUTURE TIME PERSPECTIVE QUESTIONNAIRE

QUESTIONNAIRE

December 17, 1997

Directions: This questionnaire measures your feelings or beliefs about the relationship between the here-and-now and the future. Read each statement and circle the number on the scale below each item to represent the degree to which you agree with the statement.

[On the original questionnaire, the scale below was repeated after each of the questions.]

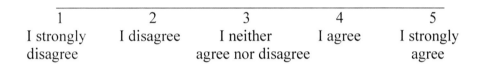

1	2	3	4	5
I strongly disagree	I disagree	I neither agree nor disagree	I agree	I strongly agree

1. What might happen to me in the long run should not be a big consideration in my making decisions now.

2. What happens to me in the long run is more important than how I feel right now.

3. In general, six months seems like a very short period of time to me.

4. As of today (December 17, 1997), June of next year seems very near.

5. I should be taking steps today to realize my future goals.

6. The most important thing in life is how I feel in the long run.

7. It's not very important to have future goals for where I might want to be in five or ten years.

8. A person should not think too much about the future.

9. Given the choice, it is better to get something I want in the future than something I want today.

10. Half a year seems like a long time to me.

11. What I do today will have little impact on what happens ten years from now.

12. It is important to have goals for where I want to be in five or ten years.

13. I don't like to plan for the future.

14. It is better to be considered a success at the end of my life than to be considered a success today.

15. Immediate pleasure is more important than what might happen in the future.

16. I find myself thinking about the future a lot.

17. Planning for the future is a waste of time.

18. Long range goals are more important than short range goals.

19. What will happen to me in the future is an important thing to consider in deciding what I should do now.

20. It often seems like the time between Rutledge weeks will never end.

21. I have been thinking a lot about what I am going to do in the future.

22. It is more important to save money for the future than to buy what I want today.

23. It's really no use worrying about the future.

24. The month of May seems a long way off.

25. Achieving my IBP's has a lot to do with achieving my long term goals.

26. For me, the time between now and New Year's Eve seems a long way off.

27. Short term goals = Long term success

28. If I reach my goals on one morning, it doesn't matter if I'm rewarded at lunchtime or at some later time in the future.

29. I can see myself one day leaving Tallangatta.

30. If you had to put a time-frame on when you'd be leaving Tallangatta, when would that be? In 1 month? 6 months? 1 yr? 5 yrs? You name it.

APPENDIX B

INTERVIEW QUESTIONS

Proposed Questions/Probes

1. Tell me about you:
    Interests, such a work, hobbies
    Family, culture
    Travel
    Education

2. Tell me about your medical problem.
    What is your diagnosis? Prognosis
    How long have you been coming to the clinic?
    How did you learn of the clinic?

3. Share, please, your treatment plan and how you think you are doing.
    Patient definition of motivation
    "Demotivation" factors
    Factors which positively influence compliance for this patient

4. Share with me the audio-visual tools you use regularly, such as video, computers, e-mail, etc.

5. Describe to me the elements that you think help a patient succeed with intervention/prevention program.
    Family support,
    Physician/healthcare worker communication
    Clinic support

6. Is there anything else you'd like to tell me about motivating you as a patient, or patients in general?

APPENDIX C

POEMS

"Life"

We all have our hard times
  going through life

The loss of a loved one,
  a broken hearted wife.

It's hard to show our feelings
It's hard to say we care

knowing when to comfort
and knowing when to share

It's just the way we say it
  that gets through the night

And it's just how we say it
that everything's alright

A word of inspiration
an understanding heart

A prayer gently spoken
  or whispered in the dark

To give your fears to Jesus
He's more than just a friend

Just give your heart to Jesus
for it to truly mend.

—Rose

Prayer for the Survivor

Almighty God, Father of mankind and Architect of the universe, hear my humble prayer.

Like so many other in this world, I have been visited by tragedy and loss. I have seen my life changed irrevocably and I have seen the consequences of my suffering exact it's toll on my family. I have also borne witness to the sufferings of others who share my pain and devastation.

I have felt anger and frustration for the circumstances that left me as I am. I have felt fear for the unknown future and what may come to pass. I have felt sorrow for the loss of my former life and the pain of my family and yes, sorrow for those who must travel where I have been and I ask Lord, that You grant me these gifts:

I ask that You grant me Your strength that my spirit may never be broken and so that the injuries to my body and soul shall someday heal and to endure what is to come.

I ask that You grant me Your wisdom that I may understand the emotions that I feel and that I can better decide for myself what course I should follow.

I ask that You grant me Your everlasting love that it may buoy my family in these troubled waters and that I may be able to love myself for who I am now.

I ask that You grant me Your tolerance that I can forgive those who cause me additional pain despite their well meaning intentions.

I ask that You to grant me Your compassion that I might aid another frightened and angry soul who suffers as I do.

I ask that You grant me Your patience Lord, for I know that the road upon which I travel is a long and difficult one.

I also ask that these gifts be given to every survivor that we may all heal and share in the bounty of life.

Father, I ask for these gifts to aid my will to endure this trial of life so that I may emerge whole. I realize that I may never be the same as I was but I have so much to give. I ask for these gifts in Jesus' name.

Amen   —Bill

It's All in Your Head

"It's all in your head," he said to me.
"You could if you wanted to, if you wanted to be
normal and fine, you could set yourself free."

"You make it worse for yourself," she said to me,
"by believing you have brain damage when there is nothing to see.
Pick yourself up by your bootstraps and get on with your life;
face it that you are normal and you'll lessen your strife."

Something was different,
but I couldn't explain.
I asked for understanding,
but got only pain.
In my extreme vulnerability I tried to belong,
but everywhere I turned I was told I was wrong.

Then one day I realized I had lost all control
and there was only one way
I knew how to be whole--
I gave them back their opinions
and validated my life,
found others like me,
brain injured for life.

One day at time
we face our real lives,
wasting no time on ignorant replies.

Honoring the truth
is to face the real me
and finally, oh finally,
I know what it is to be free.

—Mildred

APPENDIX D

QUESTIONNAIRE

MOTIVATIONAL FACTORS IN TBI RECOVERY

Motivational Factors in TBI Recovery
(Please remember that you are not required
to enter your name on this questionnaire)

I. Demographic information (circle one):

Age: 0-12   13-20   21-30   31-40   41-50   51-60   61-70   71-80   81-90   91-100

Male/Female

Ethnic Background: Spanish speaking origin   African-American   Asian   Caucasian

Other_____

Educational Level: K-6   7-12   Trade school   College

                 BA   MA   PhD   MD   JD

Other_____

Occupation prior to injury:_____

Prior to injury: Married   Single   Divorced   Widowed   Separated

Post injury: Married   Single   Divorced   Widowed   Separated

Medical insurance: Yes   No

Who was responsible for your medical bills:

     Self   Company Insurance   Workman's Comp

           Personal Insurance   Liability Insurance

Who were(are) the members of your immediate support group:

        family   friends   medical team   none

Years post injury?   0-1/2/3/4/5/6/7/8/9/10/10+

Thank you for participating in this research.

                                     Lynda G. Cleveland

Cause of injury:

car accident

bike accident

motorcycle accident

sports injury

gun shot

fall

Other_____

child abuse

assault

industrial accident

birth trauma

Circle any/all consequences you sustained as a result of your injury:

short term memory loss

long term memory loss

problems in arousal (waking)

attention

concentration

initiating activites

planning

completing actions

judgement

speech

sexual dysfunction

social skills

self-confidence

thought processing

spatial disorientation

hemiparesis (paralysis affecting one side of the body)

seizures

spasticity (stiff or awkward movements)

visual impairment

loss of taste/smell

reduced physical endurance

difficulty in sleep patterns

anxiety

depression

inappropriate behavior

outbursts/agitation

loss of social networking/feeling of isolation

other_____

How long were you in a coma?

not at all/0-24 hours/24-48 hours/3-7 days/over 7 days

Was your head injury open or closed? (circle one)

How long were you hospitalized?

not at all/observation/2 days/3-7 days/7-14 days/2 weeks-1 month/month+

How long were you in a rehabilitation facility as an in-patient?

not at all/3-7 days/7-14 days/2 weeks-1 month/ month+/year+

How long were you in a rehabilitation facility as an out-patient?

not at all/3-7 days/7-14 days/2 weeks-1 month/ month+/year+

How long did you receive care at home by a professional therapist?

not at all/3-7 days/7-14 days/2 weeks-1 month/ month+/year+

Circle all care providers that assisted you in additiona to the primary medical team and your support team:

Occupational Therapist

Physical Therapist

Respiratory Therapist

Speech Therapist

Cognitive Therapist

Vocational Therapist

What has helped you the most during rehab ?(for example, a service, or person, or tool)_____

What has helped you the least during rehab ?_____

How many years post injury did you return to work:

0-1/2/3/4/5/6/7/8/9/10/10+/have not returned

Did you return to the same job?

yes/no

I am asking you about your feelings right now looking back on your head injury and rehabilitation experience. **Please circle the extent to which you experience each feeling. Work rapidly. Your first reaction is best.**
Here is an example:

regretful 1 2 3 4 5 6 **7** (I felt extremely regretful about my experience)

regretful **1** 2 3 4 5 6 7 (I do not feel regretful about my experience at all)

Remember, 1= not at all   7= extremely

guilty		1	2	3	4	5	6	7
angry		1	2	3	4	5	6	7
depressed		1	2	3	4	5	6	7
carefree		1	2	3	4	5	6	7
elated		1	2	3	4	5	6	7
concentrating		1	2	3	4	5	6	7
drowsy		1	2	3	4	5	6	7
affectionate		1	2	3	4	5	6	7
regretful		1	2	3	4	5	6	7
dubious		1	2	3	4	5	6	7
boastful		1	2	3	4	5	6	7
active		1	2	3	4	5	6	7
defiant		1	2	3	4	5	6	7
fearful		1	2	3	4	5	6	7
playful		1	2	3	4	5	6	7
overjoyed		1	2	3	4	5	6	7
engaged in thought		1	2	3	4	5	6	7
sluggish		1	2	3	4	5	6	7
kindly		1	2	3	4	5	6	7
sad		1	2	3	4	5	6	7
skeptical		1	2	3	4	5	6	7
frustrated		1	2	3	4	5	6	7
energetic		1	2	3	4	5	6	7
rebellious		1	2	3	4	5	6	7
jittery		1	2	3	4	5	6	7
witty		1	2	3	4	5	6	7
pleased		1	2	3	4	5	6	7
intent		1	2	3	4	5	6	7
tired		1	2	3	4	5	6	7
warmhearted	1	2	3	4	5	6	7
sorry		1	2	3	4	5	6	7
suspicious		1	2	3	4	5	6	7
self-centered		1	2	3	4	5	6	7
accepting		1	2	3	4	5	6	7
grief		1	2	3	4	5	6	7
denial		1	2	3	4	5	6	7
annoyed		1	2	3	4	5	6	7

Challenge time!!!! NOW, I'm asking you to review these same adjectives and reflect upon your feelings **shortly after** your injury **(within the first 6-9 months)**. **Again, please circle the extent to which you experienced each feeling. Work rapidly. Your first reaction is best.**

Remember, 1= not at all   7= extremely

guilty		1	2	3	4	5	6	7
angry		1	2	3	4	5	6	7
depressed		1	2	3	4	5	6	7
carefree		1	2	3	4	5	6	7
elated		1	2	3	4	5	6	7
concentrating		1	2	3	4	5	6	7
drowsy		1	2	3	4	5	6	7
affectionate		1	2	3	4	5	6	7
regretful		1	2	3	4	5	6	7
dubious		1	2	3	4	5	6	7
boastful		1	2	3	4	5	6	7
active		1	2	3	4	5	6	7
defiant		1	2	3	4	5	6	7
fearful		1	2	3	4	5	6	7
playful		1	2	3	4	5	6	7
overjoyed		1	2	3	4	5	6	7
engaged in thought		1	2	3	4	5	6	7
sluggish		1	2	3	4	5	6	7
kindly		1	2	3	4	5	6	7
sad		1	2	3	4	5	6	7
skeptical		1	2	3	4	5	6	7
frustrated		1	2	3	4	5	6	7
energetic		1	2	3	4	5	6	7
rebellious		1	2	3	4	5	6	7
jittery		1	2	3	4	5	6	7
witty		1	2	3	4	5	6	7
pleased		1	2	3	4	5	6	7
intent		1	2	3	4	5	6	7
tired		1	2	3	4	5	6	7
warmhearted	1	2	3	4	5	6	7
sorry		1	2	3	4	5	6	7
suspicious		1	2	3	4	5	6	7
self-centered		1	2	3	4	5	6	7
accepting		1	2	3	4	5	6	7
grief		1	2	3	4	5	6	7
denial		1	2	3	4	5	6	7
annoyed		1	2	3	4	5	6	7

WHEW- Thank you very much for that adjective work!! You're on the home stretch....

Circle all educational tools used to assist you in recovery:

a.   One to one Instruction by:

nurse   physician   TBI survivor rehabilitation specialist

trained educator   personal support team member

b.   Group sessions

group therapy   rehabilitation agency   internet list serv TBI focus group

internet TBI chat group   community support groups

c.   Self-instruction items

written material   audio tapes   internet surfing

d.   Audio-visual tools

compact discs video tapes   interactive laser disc   computer assisted instruction

electronic mail (e-mail)   35mm slides   16 mm film

Now, in the list above place a check by any tool you did NOT have, but think might have benefited your recovery efforts.

Did you experience any problems in initial re-entry into society either in work or social activities, or volunteer efforts?
yes/no

If yes, briefly describe those problems.

THE FINAL SECTION IS ON THE NEXT PAGE!! -- Let's share our stories....
Circle your agreement with the statements of fellow TBIers:

••
" An injury to the brain, an insult to our being - ness..."

Not true of me		**True of me**			**Very true of me**			
(never felt that way)		(Agree- understand the feeling)			(Incredible description of how I feel)			
1	2	3	4	5	6	7	8	9

••

"Like living, recovery is a never-ending, ongoing process,
it's a case of learning how to live in a different body and brain."

Not true of me	**True of me**	**Very true of me**
(never felt that way)	(Agree- understand the feeling)	(Incredible description of how I feel)

1	2	3	4	5	6	7	8	9

Do I have additional burdens placed upon me from the strange maze of
medical/insurance/legal stuff? Yuk.
I am unarmed."

Not true of me	**True of me**	**Very true of me**
(never felt that way)	(Agree- understand the feeling)	(Incredible description of how I feel)

1	2	3	4	5	6	7	8	9

Yes, I am more emotional, Yes, I am angry, Yes, I am sad
But, I am no less, I just need time to remember and maybe regress,
I must mourn for who I used to be.
Give me time, give me space, don't crowd, don't demand

Not true of me	**True of me**	**Very true of me**
(never felt that way)	(Agree- understand the feeling)	(Incredible description of how I feel)

1	2	3	4	5	6	7	8	9

I want to scream, I want to shout, for the life that I lost.
I will never be like then, but I can be better

Not true of me	**True of me**	**Very true of me**
(never felt that way)	(Agree- understand the feeling)	(Incredible description of how I feel)

1	2	3	4	5	6	7	8	9

"self...for me, function and sense of self were inextricably bound together."

Not true of me	**True of me**	**Very true of me**
(never felt that way)	(Agree- understand the feeling)	(Incredible description of how I feel)

1	2	3	4	5	6	7	8	9

•••

"I wanted to scream, "HEY!, I have a brain injury, I'm not stupid!"

Not true of me   **True of me**   **Very true of me**
(never felt that way)   (Agree- understand the feeling)   (Incredible description of how I feel)

1   2   3   4   5   6   7   8   9

•••

•••

I wanted help just to be in society again.
Why don't they {rehab} teach you those survival skills?"

Not true of me   **True of me**   **Very true of me**
(never felt that way)   (Agree- understand the feeling)   (Incredible description of how I feel)

1   2   3   4   5   6   7   8   9

•••

•••

Learning compensatory skills lasts a lifetime and is empowering; waiting
to heal is not, yet the latter seems to be the focus within the medical
community, unfortunately.

Not true of me   **True of me**   **Very true of me**
(never felt that way)   (Agree- understand the feeling)   (Incredible description of how I feel)

1   2   3   4   5   6   7   8   9

•••

•••

"I can be in a room full of people and yet feel all alone."

Not true of me   **True of me**   **Very true of me**
(never felt that way)   (Agree- understand the feeling)   (Incredible description of how I feel)

1   2   3   4   5   6   7   8   9

•••

•••

I decided to finally let go of worry and fear and I now go to
church and follow the principles of the Bible.

Not true of me   **True of me**   **Very true of me**
(never felt that way)   (Agree- understand the feeling)   (Incredible description of how I feel)

1   2   3   4   5   6   7   8   9

•••

•••

I know what you mean about the writing, it does help to share it.

Not true of me   **True of me**   **Very true of me**
(never felt that way)   (Agree- understand the feeling)   (Incredible description of how I feel)

1   2   3   4   5   6   7   8   9

I will be twenty years post-injury in three weeks, and I am still recovering. I am re-learning skills, I am learning compensatory strategies, and am learning things about myself and life that I couldn't possibly have learned without the experience of the injury. I truly believe that I am a better person for experiencing this injury. I found personal strength I didn't know or believe I had, and because of that was able to love myself more than ever before.

Not true of me   **True of me**   **Very true of me**
(never felt that way)   (Agree- understand the feeling)   (Incredible description of how I feel)

1   2   3   4   5   6   7   8   9

One thing I have learned through all of this is that the world I was operating in is more messed up than I am!

Not true of me   **True of me**   **Very true of me**
(never felt that way)   (Agree- understand the feeling)   (Incredible description of how I feel)

1   2   3   4   5   6   7   8   9

I believe that the timing of rehabilitation for TBI could be altered to better the outcome for the patient.

Not true of me   **True of me**   **Very true of me**
(never felt that way)   (Agree- understand the feeling)   (Incredible description of how I feel)

1   2   3   4   5   6   7   8   9

APPENDIX E

CONCEPTUAL LABELS

Conceptual Labels

desire
self-evaluation
conversation thread
compensatory strategy
accident
improvement
money
responsibility vs. need
goal
trust in God
regret
building relationships
accomplishment
   against the odds
teaching
weight loss
follow-through
comparison to others
comparison to past
failure to identify
perception of progress
staff impressions
football
restate idea
client encouragement
interpretations for
   signatures
resist structure
awareness
self-concept
speaks Spanish to
   individualized self
staff role model
guiding conversation
"get in trouble"
frustration with staff
client focus on problem
attitude
realization

desire for home
attending the dance
questioning the system
basic skills
dislike journal
ACC
writing post-accident
coffee
coffee
coffee
value of the dollar
token vs. real money
happy equals job &
   friends
interpreting past
questioning future
radio loud
opposite sex puzzle
outgoing nature
bored at work
negotiation
task confusion
shopping organization
client interruption
grocery shopping
jealous of staff time
   with other clients
joking
laughing
laughter
remembering
   hospitalization
interior decorating skill
softball games
question age vs. ability
institutional behavior
intimidating techniques
habit
paying for the outing

vision of future
tunnel vision
obsessions
change equals negative
comfort zone
staff relations
scaffolding
receptive
language clarity
staff time
lack of explanation
vocabulary deficit
support attentiveness
   recalled
malingering
compliments vs. money
community involvement
staff warning
"I'm brain-injured"
sermon discussion
church behavior
memory tip-off
memory peg
curiosity
employment
flexibility vs
   nonflexibility
disengagement
determination
competence
wealthy not necessarily
   happy
relatedness
worker perplexed
"9 to 5"
metacognition
clarification needed
suggestions
work ethics

complaints stored up
French
assurance
staff numbers
justification
client interaction
imagination
Sarah, Sylvia, Cynthia
    Stout
multiple level
    concentration
analogies difficult
mixed conversations
dates important
preoccupied staff
privileges forgotten
staff not doing exercises
confusion on
    instructions
staff relationships
comparison
people awareness
information recognition
interpretation
people telling you "you
    can't"

testing relationships
missing home
idolizing home
dreaming of marriage
sense of humor
pick up previous
    conversation
accomplishing goals
medical knowledge
personal ideas
blank stares
time-out
client confusion

accepting "it"
impulsive
staff says not acceptable
description of goal
sequencing
uncomfortable at church
demonstrate skills
staff interpretation of
    behavior
Hallowe'en party equals
    fun
physical contact
personal conflict
freedom in community
interpretation of "lost"
recall
self triggers for anger
discussing early medical
    care
client comparisons
self doubt
remembering family
family visits
"bonzai" growth
too much trouble to
    answer

"who's on first?"
why exercise
physical sensations
unexpected changes
self-control
case manager
    relationships
organization
understanding
recalling names
spelling "Lynda"
staff/client interactions
compliments

promotion
color advancement
house responsibilities
roommate interaction
hurt in sports
one-way interaction
argument
submitting job
    applications
"I hope it's possible, not
    just hopeful"
"I can try"
"smiling face"
e-mail
FAX machine
silent signals
"that's all I hope for"
welding-out of the
    question
staff challenges
"get a life"
moving to Africa
scholarships
anger
naming the cranial
    nerves but forgetting
    your lunch
irritated
progress visualization
dreaming
competing with self
liking self
"If I can do it. You can
    do it."
self-rating
communication skills
living in the real world
people's feelings
fear
short-term goals equal
    long-term success

BIBLIOGRAPHY

Bibliography

References marked with an asterisk indicate studies cited in the text.

*Abrams, D. & Twiggs, H. (1995). Closed head injuries: The silent epidemic. Trial Diplomacy Journal, 18, 252-257.

Akridge, R. L. (1986). A community model of habilation/ rehabilitation. Journal of Rehabilitation Administration, 10, 81-87.

Allegrante, J. P., Kovar, P. A., MacKenzie, C. R., Peterson, M.G. E. & Gutin, B. (1993, Spring). A walking education program for patients with osteoarthritis of the knee: Theory and intervention strategies. Health Education Quarterly, 20(1), 63-81.

*Armstrong, C. (1991, April/May/June). Emotional changes following brain injury: Psychological and neurological components of depression, denial and anxiety. Journal of Rehabilitation, 15-21.

*Ashley, M. J. & Krych, D. K. (Eds.). (1995). Traumatic brain injury rehabilitation. Boca Raton: CRC Press, Inc.

*Atkinson, J. W. (1964). A theory of achievement motivation. In An introduction to motivation (pp. 240-268). New York: Van Nostrand.

*Babcock, D. E. & Miller, M. A. (1994). Client education: Theory & practice. St. Louis: Mosby.

Bachman, D. L. (1992). The diagnosis and management of common neurologic sequelae of closed head injury. Journal of Head Trauma Rehabilitation, 7(2), 50-59.

*Baddeley, A. (1994) The remembered self and the enacted self. In U. Neisser & R. Fivush (Eds.), The remembering self: Construction and accuracy in the self-narrative (pp. 236-242). Cambridge: Cambridge University Press.

Bame, S. I., Petersen, N. & Wray, N. P. (1993). Variation in hemodialysis patient compliance according to demographic characteristics. Social Science in Medicine, 37, 1035-1043.

Bandura, A. (1977). Social learning theory. Englewood Cliffs NJ: Prentice Hall.

*Bandura, A. (1982). Self-efficacy mechanisms in human agency. <u>American Psychologist, 37,</u> 122-147.

Bandura, A. (1987). Perceived self-efficacy: Exercise of control through self-belief. <u>Controversial issues in behavior modification. (Annual series of European Research in Behavior Therapy: 2)</u> (pp. 27-59). Alblasserdam: Swets & Seitlinger.

*Bandura, A. (1998, March). <u>Health promotion through self-efficacy.</u> Lecture presented at The Thirteenth Annual LaVerne Gallman Distinguished Lecture in Nursing, University of Texas at Austin School of Nursing.

*Bandura, A. (Ed.). (1986). <u>Social foundations of thought and action: A social cognitive theory.</u> Englewood Cliffs, NJ: Prentice Hall.

Barofsky, I. (1978). Compliance, adherence and the therapeutic alliance: Steps in the development of self-care. <u>Social Science and Medicine, 12,</u> 369-376.

Barry, P. & O'Leary, J. (1989). Roles of the psychologist on a traumatic brain injury rehabilitation team. <u>Rehabilitation Psychology, 34</u>(2), 83-90.

*Bateson, G. (1956). Communication in occupational therapy. <u>American Journal of Occupational Therapy, 10,</u> 188.

Becker, M. H. & Maiman, L. A. (1980). Strategies for enhancing patient compliance. <u>Journal of Community Health, 6,</u> 113-135.

Becker, M. H. (1979). Understanding patient compliance: The contribution of attitudes and other psychosocial factors. In S. J. Cohen (Ed.), <u>New directions in patient compliance.</u> Lexington: D. C. Heath.

Becker, M. H. (Ed.). (1974). <u>The health belief model and personal health behavior.</u> Thorofare, NJ: Charles B Slack.

*Bee, C. M. (1994, September). How to win a minor head injury case: preparation, patience, and perseverance. <u>Trial,</u> 54-57.

Ben-Sira, Z. (1986). Disability, stress and readjustment: The function of the professional's latent goals and affective behavior in rehabilitation. <u>Social Science and Medicine, 23,</u> 43-55.

*Bergland, M. M., & Thomas, K. R. (1991). Psychosocial issues following severe head injury in adolescence: Individual and family perspectives. <u>Rehabilitation Counseling Bulletin, 35,</u> 5-22.

*Berrol, S. (1986). Foreword. In Prigatano, G., <u>Neuropsychological</u> <u>rehabilitation after brain injury</u> (pp. xv-xvi). Baltimore: The John Hoplins University Press

Berry, B. (1998, January). Personal Interview with the author.

Bleiberg, J., Cope, D. N. & Spector, J. (1989, February). Cognitive assessment and therapy in traumatic brain injury. <u>Physical Medicine and</u> <u>Rehabilitation, 3</u>(1), 95-120.

*Bloom, M. (1987, Fall/Winter). Toward a technology in primary prevention: Educational strategies and tactics. <u>Journal of Primary Prevention. 8</u> (1 & 2), NEED pages

*Bogdan, R. C. & Biklen, S. K. (1992). <u>Qualitative research for education: An</u> <u>introduction to theory and methods</u>. (2nd ed.). Boston: Allyn & Bacon.

*Bolles, R. C. (1975). <u>Theory of motivation</u> (2nd ed.). New York: Harper & Row.

*Bond, M. R. (1990). Standardized methods of assessing and predicting outcome. In M. Rosenthal, M.R.Bond & J. R. Miller (Eds.), <u>Rehabilitation of the</u> <u>head injured adult</u> (2nd ed., pp. 97-113). Philadelphia: F. A. Davis.

*Bontke, C. (1990). Medical advances in the treatment of brain injury. In J. S. Kreutzer & P. Wehman (Eds.), <u>Community integration following</u> <u>traumatic brain injury</u> (Chapter 1). Baltimore, MD: Paul Brookes Publishing Company.

Borich, G. D. & Jemelka, R. P. (1982). <u>Programs and systems: An evaluation</u> <u>perspective</u>. New York: Academic Press.

*Brennan, P. F., Ripich, S. & Moore, S. M. (1991). The use of home-based computers to support persons living with AIDS/ARC. <u>Journal of</u> <u>Community Health Nursing, 8</u>(1), 3-14.

*Brennan, P. F., Moore, K S. M., Smyth, K. A. (1992). Alzheimer's disease caregivers' uses of a computer network. <u>Western Journal of Nursing</u> <u>Research, 14</u>(5), 662-673.

Brock, D. W. & Wartman, S. A. (1990). When competent patients make irrational choices. <u>New England Journal of Medicine, 322,</u> 1595-1599.

*Brooks, D. (1976). Long- and short-term memory in head injured patients. Cortex, 11, 329-340.

*Browning, R. A. (1995). Neurotransmitters and pharmacology. In M. J. Ashley & D. Krych (Eds.), Traumatic brain injury rehabilitation (pp. 67-119). Boca Raton: CRC Press.

*Bruner, J. (1994). The "remembered" self. In U. Neisser & R. Fivush (Eds.), The remembering self: Construction and accuracy in the self-narrative (pp. 41-54). Cambridge: Cambridge University Press.

Buck, R. (1988). Human motivation and emotion. (2nd ed.). New York: John Wiley & Sons.

*Cahn, G. (1996). Traumatic brain injury: Understanding memory impairment. Trial Diplomacy Journal, 19, 101-108.

*Cahn, G. (1997). Traumatic brain injuries: Personality impairments and their importance. Trial Diplomacy Journal, 20, 25-33.

*Cameron, R. & Best, J. A. (1987). Promoting adherence to health behavior change interventions: Recent findings from behavioral research. Patient Education and Counseling, 10, 139-154.

Carlson, J. G. & Hatfield, E. (1992). Psychology of emotion. Fort Worth: Harcourt Brace Jovanovich College Publishers.

*Charlton, W. (1987). Weakness of the will. London: Blackwell.

Charmaz, K. (1990). 'Discovering' chronic illness: Using grounded theory. Social Science Medicine, 30(11) 1161-1172.

*Chittum, W. R., Johnson, K., Chittum, J. M., Guercio, J. M. & McMorrow, M. J. (1996). Road to awareness: An individualized training package for increasing knowledge and comprehension of personal deficits in persons with acquired brain injury. Brain Injury, 10(10), 763-776.

*Cicerone, K. D. (1989). Psychotherapeutic interventions with traumatically brain-injured patients. Rehabilitation Psychology, 34(2), 105-114.

*Cleveland, L. G. & Taylor, S. A. (1985). Detour ahead!: Wit and wisdom in life's crises. Melbourne, Australia: Living Promotions, Pty. Ltd.

Condeluci, A., Cooperman, S. & Seif, B. A. (1987). Social role valorization: A model for community reentry. <u>Journal of Head Trauma Rehabilitation,</u> <u>2</u>(1), 49-56.

*Connell, J. P. (1990). Context, self, and action: A motivational analysis of self-system processes across the life-span. In D. Cicchetti (Ed.), <u>The self in</u> <u>transition: From infancy to childhood</u> (pp. 61-97). Chicago: University of Chicago Press.

*Connell, J. P. & Wellborn, J. G. (1991). Competence, autonomy, and relatedness: A motivational analysis of self-system processes. In M. R. Gunnar & L. A. Sroufe (Eds.), <u>Minnesota symposium on child</u> <u>psychology: Vol. 23. Self processes in development</u> (pp. 167-216). Hillsdale, NJ: Lawrence Erlbaum.

Cordova, D. I. & Lepper, M. R. (1996). Intrinsic motivation and the process of learning: Beneficial effects of contextualization, personalization, and choice. <u>Journal of Educational Psychology, 88</u>(4), 715-730.

*Corno, L. (1993, March). The best-laid plans: Modern conceptions of volition and educational research. <u>Educational Researcher, 22</u>(2), 14-22.

Corno, L. (1997). Motivation, volition, and collaborative innovation in classroom literacy . In J. T. Guthrie & A. Wigfield (Eds.), <u>Promoting literacy</u> <u>engagement: Motivational, strategic reading through integrated instruction</u> (pp. 51-67). Newark, DL: International Reading Association.

Corno, L. & Jackson, D., III. (1996). Individual differences in affective and conative functions. In D. C. Berliner & R. C. Calfee (Eds.), <u>Handbook of</u> <u>educational psychology</u> (pp. 243-310). New York: Simon & Schuster Macmillan.

*Cramer, J. (1991a). Overview of methods to measure and enhance patient compliance. In J. A. Cramer & B. Spilker (Eds.), <u>Patient compliance in</u> <u>medical and clinical trials</u> (pp. 3-10). New York: Raven Press, Ltd.

*Cramer, J. A. (1991b). Identifying and improving compliance patterns. <u>Patient</u> <u>compliance in medical practice and clinical trials</u> (pp. 387-392). New York: Raven Press, Ltd.

*Cramer, J. A. & Spilker, B. (Eds.). (1991). <u>Patient compliance in medical</u> <u>practice and clinical trials</u>. New York: Raven Press.

Cripe, L. (1989). Neurological and psychosocial assessment of the brain -injured person: Clinical concepts and guidelines. <u>Rehabilitation Psychology,</u> <u>34</u>(2), 93-100.

Cripe, L. I. (1989). Neuropsychological and psychosocial assessment of the brain-injured person: Clinical concepts and guidelines. <u>Rehabilitation</u> <u>Psychology, 34</u>(2), 93-103.

*Crisp, R. (1992, October/November/December). Return to work after traumatic brain injury. <u>Journal of Rehabilitation, 58</u>(4), 27-33.

*Crisp, R. (1994, Winter). Social reintegration after traumatic brain impairment: a qualitative analysis. <u>Journal of Applied Rehabilitation Counseling,</u> <u>25</u>(4), 16-20.

Cromer, B. A. (1991). Behavioral strategies to increase compliance in adolescents. <u>Patient compliance in medical practice and clinical trials</u> (pp. 99-105). New York: Raven Press, Ltd.

*Csikszentmihalyi, M. (1990). <u>Flow: The psychology of optimal experience.</u> New York: Harper Perennial.

Daltroy, L. H. & Liang, M. H. (1993, Spring). Arthritis education: Opportunities and state of the art. <u>Health Education Quarterly, 20</u>(1), 3-16.

*Damrosch, S. (1991, December). General strategies for motivating people to change their behavior. <u>Nursing Clinics of North America, 26</u>(4), 833-843.

Dann, M. D. (1984). Loss of self. <u>Cognitive Rehabilitation, 2</u>(6), 11.

*Davies, P. (1979). Motivation, responsibility and sickness in the psychiatric treatment of alcoholism. <u>Journal of Psychiatry, 134,</u> 449-458.

*Davies, P. M. (1994). <u>Starting again: Early rehabilitation after traumatic brain</u> <u>injury or other severe brain lesion</u> (p. 19). New York: Springer-Verlag.

*Davis, E. M. (1990, November). Mild to moderate brain injury: A silent epidemic. <u>Trial,</u> 109-114.

Davis, M. S. (1968). Variations in patients' compliance with doctors' advice: An empirical analysis of patterns of communication. <u>American Journal of</u> <u>Public Health, 58,</u> 284.

*Deardorff, W. W. (1986, Spring). Computerized health education: a comparison with traditional formats. Health Education Quarterly, 13(1), 61-72.

*DeBeaugrande, R., & Dressler, W. (1981). Introduction to text linguistics. New York: Longman.

*Deci, E. L. (1975). Intrinsic motivation. New York: Plenum Press.

*Deci, E. L. & Ryan, R. (1980). The empirical exploration of intrinsic motivational processes. Advances in experimental psychology, Volume 13 (pp. 40-77). New York: Academic Press, Inc.

*Deci, E. L. & Ryan, R. M. (1985). Intrinsic motivation and self-determination in human behavior. New York: Plenum Press.

*Deci, E. L. & Ryan, R. M. (1991). A motivational approach to self: Integration in personality. In R. Dienstbier (Ed.), Nebraska symposium on motivation: Vol. 38. Perspectives on motivation (pp. 237-288). Lincoln: University of Nebraska Press.

*Deci, E. L., Vallerand, R. J., Pelletier, L. G., & Ryan, R. M. (1991). Motivation in education: The self-determination perspective. Educational Psychologist, 26, 325-346.

DeJong, G., Batavia, A. I. & Williams, J. M. (1990). Who is responsible for the lifelong well-being of a person with a head injury? Journal of Head Trauma Rehabilitation, 5(1), 9-22.

Derryberry, D. & Tucker, D. M. (1992). Neural mechanisms of emotion. Journal of Consulting and Clinical Psychology, 60, 329-338.

*Dewey, J. (1934). Art as experience. New York: Minton, Balch.

DiMatteo, M. R. & DiNicola, D. D. (1982). Achieving patient compliance: The psychology of the medical practitioner's role. New York: Pergamon.

*Eccles, J. (1983). Expectancies, values and academic behaviors. In J. T. Spence (Ed.), Achievement and achievement motives (pp. 75-146). San Francisco: Freeman.

*Edelstein, B. A. & Couture, E. T. (Eds.). (1983). Behavioral assessment and rehabilitation of the traumatically brain-damaged. New York: Plenum Press.

*Ellerd, D., Moore, S. C., Speer, D. & Lackey, R. K. (1994). Nontraditional supports in supported employment: Preliminary results for persons with traumatic brain injury. Journal of Applied Rehabilitation Counseling, 25(4), 22-25.

*Emanuel, E. J. & Emanuel, L. L. (1992). Four models of the physician-patient relationship. Journal of the American Medical Association, 267(16), 2221-2226.

*Engelhardt, H. T., Jr. (1977). Defining occupational therapy: The meaning of therapy and the virtues of occupation. American Journal of Occupational Therapy, 31, 666-672.

Eraker, S. A., Kirscht, J. P. & Becker, M. H. (1984). Understanding and improving patient compliance. Annals of Internal Medicine, 100, 258-268.

*Erlandson, D. A., Harris, E. L., Skipper, B. L. & Allen, S. D. (1993). Doing naturalistic inquiry: A guide to methods. Newbury Park, CA: SAGE Publications.

Evans, P., Haffey, W. J. & Cope, D. N. (1990). Treatment of behavioral disorders. In M. Rosenthal & E. R. Griffith (Eds.), Rehabilitation of the Adult and Child with Traumatic Brain Injury (2nd ed., pp. 179-192). Philadelphia: F A Davis.

Fabiano, R. J. & Goran, D. A. (1992). A principal component analysis of the katz adjustment scale in a traumatic brain injury rehabilitation sample. Rehabilitation Psychology, 37(2), 75-85.

Falconer, J. (1996). Head injuries happen to families. [On-line] Available Internet: Brain Train.

Falconer, J. (1997). Cognitive-behavioral head injury rehabilitation. [On-line] Available Internet: Brain Train.

Falconer, J. (1998, January). Personal Interview with the author.

Falconer, J. & Tercilla, E. (Rehabilitation Psychology Associates - Brain Train.) Living with head injury: Post-rehabilitation recovery. [On-line] Available Internet: Brain Train.

Falvo, D. R. (1991). Medical and psychosocial aspects of chronic illness and disability. Gaithersburg, MD: Aspen Publishers, Inc.

*Falvo, D. R. (1994). <u>Effective patient education: A guide to increased compliance</u> (2nd ed). Gaithersburg, MD: Aspen Publishers, Inc.

Fein, L. D. (Ed.). (1988). <u>The exceptional brain</u>. . New York: The Guilford Press.

Feldman, R. S. (Ed.). (1992). <u>Applications of nonverbal behavioral theories and research</u>. Hillsdale, NJ: Lawrence Erlbaum Associates, Publishers.

*Fleming, J. M., Strong, J. & Ashton, R. (1996). Self-awareness of deficits in adults with traumatic brain injury: How best to measure? <u>Brain Injury, 10</u>(1), 1-15.

*Fordyce, D., Roueche, J. & Prigatano, G. (1983). Enhanced emotional reactions in chronic head trauma patients. <u>Journal of Neurology, Neurosurgery, and Psychiatry, 46</u>, 620-624.

*Frankl, V. E. (1984). <u>Man's search for meaning</u> (3rd ed). New York: Simon & Schuster, Inc.

Fraser, R. T. (1991). Vocational evaluation. <u>Journal of Head Trauma, 6</u>(3), 46-58.

*Fraser, R. T., Clemmons, D. C. & McMahon, B. T. (1990). Vocational rehabilitation counseling. In J. S. Kreutzer & C. F. Wehman (Eds.), <u>Community integration following traumatic brain injury</u> (pp. 169-184). Baltimore: Paul H. Brooks.

*Freed, R. C., & Broadhead, G. J. (1989). Discourse communities, sacred texts, and institutional norms. <u>College Composition and Communication, 38</u>, 154-165

Freedman, P., Bleiberg, J. & Freedland, K. (1987). Anticipatory behavior deficits in closed head injury. <u>Journal of Neurology, Neurosurgery, and Psychiatry, 50</u>, 398-401.

*Fugate, L. P., Spacek, L. A., Kresty, L. A. & Mysiw, W. J. (1997a, September). Measurement and treatment of agitation following traumatic brain injury: II. A survey of the Brain Injury Special Interest Group of the American Academy of Physical Medicine and Rehabilitation. <u>Archives of Physical Medicine and Rehabilitation, 78</u>, 924-928.

*Fugate, L. P., Spacek, L. A., Kresty, L. A., Levy, C. E. & Mysiw, W. J. (1997b, September). Definition of agitation following traumatic brain injury: I. A survey of the Brain Injury Special Interest Group of the American Academy of Physical Medicine and Rehabilitation. <u>Archives of Physical Medicine and Rehabilitation, 78,</u> 917-923.

Garske, G. G. & Thomas, K. R. (1992, September). Self-reported self-esteem and depression: Indexes of psychosocial adjustment following severe traumatic brain injury. <u>Rehabilitation Counseling Bulletin, 36</u>(1), 44-52.

Geelen, R. J. G. M. & Soons, P. H. G. M. (1996). Rehabilitation: An 'everyday' motivation model. <u>Patient Education and Counseling, 28,</u> 69-77.

*Gergen, K. J., & Gergen, M. M. (1988). Narrative and the self as relationship. In L. Berkowitz (Ed.), <u>Advances in experimental social psychology,</u> (pp. 17-56). San Diego: Academic Press.

*Glasser, L. B. &. Strauss, A. (1967). <u>The discovery of grounded theory: Strategies for qualitative research.</u> Chicago: Aldine.

*Golden, C. J., Moses, J. A., Coffman, J. A., Miller, W. R. & Strider, F. D. (1983). <u>Clinical neuropsychology: Interface with neurologic and psychiatric disorders.</u> Orlando: Grune & Stratton, Inc. (Harcourt Brace Jovanovich, Publishers).

*Goldstein, K. (1952). The effect of brain damage on the personality. <u>Psychiatry, 15,</u> 245-260.

*Graham, D. L., Adams, J. H. & Doyle, D. (1978). Ischemic brain damage in fatal nonmissile head injuries. <u>Journal of Neurological Sciences, 39,</u> 213-234.

*Graham, O. & Schubert, W. (1985). A model for developing and pre-testing a multimedia teaching program to enhance the self-care behavior of diabetes insipidus patients. <u>Patient Education and Counseling, 7,</u> 53-64.

*Green, C. A. (1987). What can patient health education coordinators learn from ten years of compliance research? <u>Patient Education and Counseling, 10,</u> 167-174.

*Grice, H. P. (1975). Logic and conversation. In P. Cole & J. L. Morgan (Eds.) <u>Syntax and semantics: Speech acts </u>(Vol. 3, pp. 41-56). New York: Academic Press.

Grieco, A., Garnett, S. A., Glassman, K. S., Valoon, P. L. & McClure, M. L. (1990). New York University Medical Center's Cooperative Care Unit:

Patient education and family participation during hospitalization - The first ten years. Patient Education and Counseling, 15, 3-15.

Griffith, E. & Rosenthal, M. (Eds.). (1990). Rehabilitation of the adult and child with traumatic brain injury. Philadelphia: F. A. Davis.

Grigsby, J. (1986). Depersonalization following minor closed head injury. The International Journal of Clinical Neuropsychology, 8(2), 65-68.

*Guba, E. G. & Lincoln, Y. S. (1981). Effective evaluation. San Francisco: Jossey-Bass Publishers.

*Guba, E. G., & Lincoln, Y. S. (1989). Fourth generation evaluation. Newbury Park, CA: SAGE.

Haaland, K. (1992). Introduction to the Special Section on the Emotional Concomitants of Brain Damage. Journal of Counsulting and Clinical Psychology, 60(3), 327-328.

*Haffey, W. J. & Lewis, F. D. (1989). Programming for occupational outcomes following traumatic brain injury. Rehabilitation Psychology, 34(2), 147-158.

*Hagner, D. C., & Helm, D. T. (1994). Qualitative methods in rehabilitation research. Rehabilitation Counseling Bulletin, 37, 290-303.

Hall, K., Hamilton, B., Gordon, W. & Zasler, N. (1993). Characteristics and comparisons of functional assessment indices: Disability Rating Scale, Functional Independence Measure, and Functional Assessment Measure. Journal of Head Trauma Rehabilitation, 8(2), 60-74.

*Harter, S. (1981). A model of mastery motivation in children. In W. A. Collins (Ed.), Aspects on the development of competence: The Minnesota symposia on child psychology, 14 (p. 218). Hillsdale, NJ: Lawrence Erlbaum Associates, Inc.

*Haynes, R. B., Sackett, D. L. & Taylor, D. W. (Eds.). (1979). Compliance in health care. Baltimore: John Hopkins University Press.

Heilman, K. & Watson, R. (1991). Intentional motor disorders. Frontal lobe function and dysfunction (pp. 208-209). New York: Oxford University Press.

*Heilman, K. M. & Valenstein, E. (Eds.). (1993). Clinical neuropsychology (3rd ed.). New York: Oxford University Press.

*Helfrich, C., & Kielhofner. (1993, April). Volitional narratives and the meaning of therapy. American Journal of Occupational Therapy, 48(4), 319-326.

*Helfrich, C., Kielhofner, G. & Mattingly, C. (1994). Volition as narrative: Understanding motivation in chronic illness. American Journal of Occupational Therapy, 48, 311-317.

Helm, D. T. & Hagner, D. C. (1994, June). Qualitative methods in rehabilitation research. Rehabilitation Counseling Bulletin, 37(4), 290-301.

*Hewison, A. (1995). Nurses' power in interactions with patients. Journal of Advanced Nursing, 21, 75-82.

*Hirst, W. (1994). The remembered self in amnesics. In U. Neisser & R. Fivush (Eds.), The remembering self: Construction and accuracy in the self-narrative (pp. 252-277). Cambridge: Cambridge University Press.

*Holmes, B. C. (1996). Negotiation of meaning in physician-patient communication during cancer treatment. Unpublished doctoral dissertation, University of Texas, Austin.

Holms, G. E. & Karst, R. H. (1990). The institutionalization of disability myths: Impact on vocational rehabilitation services. Journal of Rehabillitation, 56(1), 20-27.

*Holt, E. B. (1915). The Freudian wish and its place in ethics. New York: Holt.

Horowitz, L. (1985, February). The self-care motivation model: Theory and practice in healthy human development. Journal of School Health, 55(2), 57-61.

Hoskins, M. & Leseho, J. (January/February, 1996). Changing metaphors of the self: Implications for counseling. Journal of Counseling & Development, 74, 243-251.

Howard, D. & Hatfield, F. M. (1987). Aphasia therapy: Historical and contemporary issues. East Sussex, U.K.: Lawrence Erlbaum Associates, Ltd.

*Howard, M. (1998, January). Personal Interview with the author.

*Husman, J. (1998, January). Personal Interview with the author.

*Irwin, C. E., Millstein, S., & Ellen, J. M. (1993, July). Appointment-keeping behavior in adolescents: Factors associated with follow-up appointment-keeping. Pediatrics, 92(1), 20-23.

*Janz, N. & Becker, M. (1984). The health belief model: A decade later. Health Education Quarterly, 11, 1-47.

*Jenny, J. (1983, September-October). A compliance model for diabetic instruction. Rehabilitation Literature, 44(9-10), 258-263.

Johnson, C. N. (1990). If you had my brain, where would I be?: Children's understanding of brain and identity. Child Development, 61, 962-972.

*Kaplan, S. P. (1993). Five-year tracking of psychosocial changes in people with severe traumatic brain injury. Rehabilitation Counseling Bulletin, 36, 151-159.

*Karpman, T., Wolfe, S. & Vargo, J. W. (1986). The psychological adjustment of adult clients and their parents following closed-head injury. Journal of Applied Rehabilitation Counseling, 17, 28-33.

Kasl, S. V. (1975). Issues in patient adherence to health care regimens. Journal of Human Stress, 1, 5-17.

Kaufman, B. N. (1994). Son-rise: The miracle continues. Tiburon, CA: H. J. Kramer, Inc.

Keany, K. C. M. & Glueckauf, R. I. (1993). Disability and value change: An overview and reanalysis of acceptance of loss theory. Rehabilitation Psychology and Work Adjustment Bulletin, 15, 57-64.

Kielhofner, G. (1985). A model of human occupation. Theory and application. Baltimore: Williams & Wilkins.

Kielhofner, G. (1994, April). Volitional narratives and the meaning of therapy. The American Journal of Occupational Therapy, 48(4), 319-326.

*Kim, M. Y. (1995, Winter). A multimedia information system for home health-care support. Multimedia at Work, pp. 83-87.

Klein, G. S. (1970). Perception, Motives, and Personality. New York: Alfred A Knopf.

*Kleinginna, P. R. & Kleinginna, A. M. (1981). A categorized list of motivitation definitions, with a suggestion for a consensual definition. <u>Motivation and Emotion, 5,</u> 263-291.

*Klinger, E. (1975, January). Consequences of commitment to and disengagement from incentives. <u>Psychological Review, 82</u>(1), 1-25.

*Klonoff, P. S., O'Brien, K. P., Prigatano, G. P., Chiapello, D. A. & Cunningham, M. (1989). Cognitive retraining after traumatic brain injury and its role in facilitating awareness. <u>Journal of Head Trauma Rehabilitation, 4</u>(3), 37-45.

*Kosslyn, S. M. & Koenig, O. (1992). <u>Wet mind: The new cognitive neuroscience.</u> New York: The Free Press.

*Kraus, J. F. & Sorenson, S. B. (1994). Epidemiology. In J. M. Silver, S. C. Yudofsky & R. E. Hales (Eds.), <u>Neuropsychiatry of traumatic brain injury</u> (pp. 3-41). Washington, DC: American Psychiatric Press.

Kraus, J., Black, M., Hessol, N., Ley, P., Rokan, W., Sullivan, C., Bowers, S., Knowlton & Marshall, L. (1983). The incidence of acute brain injury and serious impairment in a defined population. <u>American Journal of Epidemiology, 119,</u> 186-201.

*Krefting, L. (1990). Double bind and disability: The case of traumatic head injury. <u>Social Science and Medicine, 30,</u> 859-865.

*Kress, G. (1989). <u>Linguistic processes in sociocultural practice.</u> Oxford, England: Oxford University Press.

*Kreutzer, J. S. & Wehman, P. (Eds.). (1990). <u>Community integration following traumatic brain injury.</u> Baltimore: Paul H Brookes Publishing Co., Inc.

*Kreutzer, J. S., Gordon, W. A. & Wehman, P. (1989). Cognitive Remediation following traumatic brain injury. <u>Rehabilitation Psychology, 34</u>(2), 117-133.

Kuhl, J. & Blankenship, V. (1979). The dynamic theory of achievement motivation: From episodic to dynamic thinking. <u>Psychological Review, 86</u>(2), 141-151.

*Kuzel, A. J. (n.d.). <u>Health promotion/disease prevention within the doctor-patient relationship.</u> Unpublished funding proposal. Richmond, VA: National Fund for Medical Education.

Lam, C. S., Priddy, D. A. & Johnson, P. (1991). Neuropsychological indicators of employability following traumtaic brain injury. <u>Rehabilitation Counseling Bulletin, 35</u>, 68-74.

Lazarus, R. S. (1987). Constructs of the mind in mental health and psychotherapy. In J. Dauwalder & M. P. V. Hobi (Eds.), <u>Controversial issues in behavior modification. (Annual series of European Research in Behavior Therapy: 2)</u> (pp. 11-26). Alblasserdam: Swets & Zeitlinger.

*Leland, M., Lewis, F. D., Hinman, S. & Carrillo, R. (1988, June). Functional retraining of traumatically brain injured adults in a transdisciplinary environment. <u>Rehabilitation Counseling Bulletin, 31</u>, 289-297.

*Lepper, M. R., & Greene, D. (1978). <u>The hidden costs of reward: New perspectives on the psychology of human motivation.</u> Hillsdale, NJ: Erlbaum.

*Lepper, M. R., Greene, D., & Nisbett, R. E. (1973). Undermining children's intrinsic interest with extrinic rewards: A test of the overjustification hypothesis. <u>Journal of Personality and Social Psychology, 28,</u> 129-137.

*Levin, H. S., Benton, H. S. & Grossman, R. G. (1983). <u>Neurobehavioral consequences of closed head injury.</u> New York: Oxford University Press.

*Levin, H. S., Eisenberg, H. M. & Benton, A. L. (Eds.). (1991). <u>Frontal lobe function and dysfunction.</u> New York: Oxford University Press.

*Lewin, K. (1935). <u>A dynamic theory of personality.</u> New York: McGraw-Hill.

*Lincoln, Y. S. (1992, November). Sympathetic connections between qualitative methods and health research. <u>Qualitative Health Research, 2</u>(4), 375-391.

*Lincoln, Y. S. & Guba, E. G. (1985). <u>Naturalistic inquiry.</u> Beverly Hills, CA: SAGE Publications, Inc.

Linge, F. R. (1990). Faith, hope and love: Nontraditional therapy in recovery from serious head injury, A personal account. <u>The Canadian Journal of Psychology, 44,</u> 116-129.

Long, C. J., Cullen, F. T., Frank, J. & Wozniak, J. F. (1984). A model of recovery for the total rehabilitation of individuals with head trauma. <u>Journal of Rehabilitation, 50</u>(1), 39-45, 70.

*Loring, K. (1996). <u>Patient education, a practical approach</u>. Thousand Oaks, CA: SAGE Publications, Inc.

Mallik, K. (1990). Rehabilitation engineering and environmental modifications. In P. Wehman & J. S. Kreutzer (Eds.), <u>Vocational Rehabilitation for Persons with Traumatic Brain Injury</u> (pp. 89-104). Rockville, MD: Aspen.

*Mandleberg, I. (1975). Cognitive recovery after severe head injury. <u>Journal of Neurology, Neurosurgery and Psychiatry, 38,</u> 1127-1132.

Marzuk, P. M. (1945). The right kind of paternalism. <u>New England Journal of Medicine, 313,</u> 1474-1476.

Maslow, A. H. (1971). <u>The farther reaches of human nature</u>. New York: The Viking Press.

Mattingly, C. (1994, April). Volition as narrative: Understanding motivation in chronic illness. <u>The American Journal of Occupational Therapy, 48</u>(4), 311-317.

Mattis, P. J., Hannay, H. J., Plenger, P. M. & Pollock, L. (1994, July). Head injury and the Satz-Mogel type short form WAIS-R. <u>Journal of Clinical Psychology, 50</u>(4), 605-614.

*Maultsby, M. C., Jr., & Hendricks, A. (1974). <u>You and your emotions</u>. Appleton, WI: Rational Self-Help Books.

McMahon, B. T. & Fraser, R. T. (1988). Basic issues and trends in head injury rehabilitation. In S. E. Rubin & N. M. Rubin (Eds.), <u>Contemporary Challenges to the Rehabilitation Counseling Profession</u> (pp. 147-215). Baltimore, MD: Paul H. Brooks.

*Meece, J. L. & Holt, K. (1993). A pattern analysis of students' achievement goals. <u>Journal of Educational Psychology, 85</u>(4), 582-590.

*<u>Merriam-Webster's collegiate dictionary</u> (10th ed). (1993). Springfield, MA: Merriam-Webster.

*Meyer, D. K. (1993). What is scaffolded instruction? Definitions, distinguishing features, and misnomers. In D. J. Leu & C. K. Kinzer (Eds.), <u>Examining central issues in literacy research, theory, and practice: 42nd Yearbook of the National Reading Conference</u> (pp. 41-53). Chicago, IL: The National Reading Conference, Inc.

*Mikhail, B. (1981, October). The health belief model: A review and critical evaluation of the model, research, and practice. Advances in Nursing Science, 65-82.

Millis, S. R. (1994, July). Assessment of motivation and memory with the Recognition Memory Test after fincially compensable mild head injury. Journal of Clinical Psychology, 50(4), 601-604.

Morisky, D. E., Malotte, C. K., Choi, P., Davidson, P., Rigler, S., Sugland, B. & Langer, M. (1990, Fall). A patient education program to improve adherence rates with antituberculosis drug regimens. Health Education Quarterly, 17(3), 253-267.

*Mullinax, C. H. (1995, Mar/Apr). Cardiac rehabilitation programs and the problem of patient dropout. Rehabilitation Nursing, 20(2), 90-92.

*Neisser, U. (1994) Self-narratives: True and false. In U. Neisser & R. Fivush (Eds.), The remembering self: Construction and accuracy in the self-narrative (pp.1-18). Cambridge: Cambridge University Press.

*Neisser, U., & Fivush, R. (Eds.). (1994). Remembering self: Construction and accuracy in the self-narrative. New York: W. W. Norton & Company.

Nelson, L. D. & Cicchetti, D. V. (1995). Assessment of emotional functioning in brain-impaired individuals. Psychological Assessment, 7(3), 404-413.

*Nemeth, A. J. (1988). Litigating head trauma: The "hidden" evidence of disability. American Journal of Trial Advocacy, 12, 239-272.

*Ninomiya, J., Ashley, M., Raney, M., Krych, D. (1995). Case management of brain injury: An overview. In M. J. Ashley & D. K. Krych (Eds.), Traumatic brain injury rehabilitation (pp. 367-396). Boca Raton: CRC Press.

*Noble, D. N. & Hamilton, A. K. (1983, November/December). Coping and complying: A challenge in health care. Social Work, 462-466.

*Nochi, M. (1997). Loss of self: A narrative study on people with traumatic brain injuries . Unpublished doctoral dissertation, Syracuse University.

*Norman, D. (1990). The design of everyday things. New York: Doubleday.

*Northouse, P. G. & Northouse, L. L. (1992). Health communication: Strategies for health professionals (2nd ed). Norwalk, CT: Appleton & Lange.

*Nuttin, J. & Lens, W. (1985). <u>Future time perspective and motivation</u>. Leuven, Belgium, and Hillsdale, NJ: Leuven University Press and Lawrence Erlbaum Associates.

*Olney, M. F. & Salomone, P. R. (1992, Fall).   Empowerment and choice in supported employment: Helping people to help themselves. <u>Journal of Applied Rehabilitation, 23</u>(3), 41-44.

*Ostwald, S. (1989). An overview of rehabilitation consideration for persons with head injuries. <u>Journal of Applied Rehabilitation Counseling, 22</u>(4), 22-26.

*Owens, N. J., Larrat, E. P. & Fretwell, M. D. (1991). Improving compliance in the older patient: The role of comprehensive functional assessment. In J. A. Cramer & B. Spilker (Eds.), <u>Patient Compliance in Medical Practice and Clinical Trials</u> (pp. 107-119). New York: Raven Press, Ltd.

*Parker, R. S. (1990).   <u>Traumatic brain injury and neuropsychological impairment</u>. New York: Springer-Verlag.

Parsons, O. A. & Prigatano, G. P. (1978).   Methodological considerations in clinical neuropsychological research. <u>Journal of Consulting and Clinical Psychology, 46</u>(4), 608-619.

*Patton, M. Q. (1990).   <u>Qualitative evaluation and research methods</u> (2nd ed). Newbury Park, CA: SAGE Publications, Inc.

*Pender, N. (1975). A conceptual model for preventive health behavior. <u>Nursing Outlook, 23,</u> 385-391.

*Persinger, M. A. (1993). Personality changes following brain injury as a grief response to the loss of self: Phenomenological themes as indices of local lability and neurocognitive structuring as psychotherapy. <u>Psychological Reports, 72,</u> 1059-1068.

*Petri, H. L. (1991). <u>Motivation: Theory, research, and applications</u> (3rd ed.). Belmont, CA: Wadsworth Publishing Company.

*Petzel, S., Ellis, L. B., Budd, J. R., Johnson, Y. (1992). Microcomputers for behavioral health education: Developing and evaluating patient education for the chronically ill. <u>Computer applications in mental health</u> (pp. 167-183). MN: The Haworth Press, Inc.

Pfeiffer, D. (1993). Overview of the disability movement: History, legislative record, and political implications. <u>Policy Studies Journal, 21,</u> 724-31.

Pintrich, P. R. & Schunk, D. H. (1996). <u>Motivation in education: Theory, research, and applications</u>. Englewood Cliffs, New Jersey: Prentice-Hall, Inc.

*Pommier, B. (1992, March-April). Factors affecting learning in a coronary artery disease rehabilitation class. <u>Rehabilitation Nursing, 17</u>(2), 64-67.

Ponsford, J. (1995). <u>Traumatic brain injury: Rehabilitation for everyday adaptive living</u>. Hove, UK: Lawrence Erlbaum.

*Prawat, R. S. & Floden, R. E. (1994). Philosophical perspectives on constructivist views of learning. <u>Educational Psychologist, 29,</u> 37-48.

Pribram, K. H. (1985). Subdivisions of the frontal cortex. In E. Perecman (Ed.), <u>The frontal lobes revisited</u>. Hillsdale, New Jersey: Lawrence Erlbaum Associates.

*Prigatano, G. (1978). Awareness of deficit after brain injury. In S. Fingers (Ed.), <u>Recovery from brain injury</u> (p. 348). New York: Plenum Press.

*Prigatano, G. (1996). Behavioral limitations TBI patients tend to underestimate: A replication and extension with lateralized cerebral dysfunction. <u>The Clinical Neuropsychologist, 10</u>(2), 191-201.

*Prigatano, G. P. (1986). <u>Neuropsychological rehabilitation after brain injury</u>. Baltimore, MD: The John Hopkins University Press.

Prigatano, G. P. (1987). Personality and psychosocial consequences after brain injury. In M. J. Meier & L. Diller (Eds.), <u>Neuropsychological Rehabilitation</u> (pp. 355-378). New York: Churchill Livingstone.

Prigatano, G. P. (1987). Recovery and cognitive retraining after craniocerebral trauma. <u>Journal of Learning Disabilities, 20</u>(10), 603-613.

*Prigatano, G. P. (1989a). Bring it up in milieu: Toward effective traumatic brain injury rehabilitation interaction. <u>Rehabilitation Psychology, 34</u>(2), 135-144.

*Prigatano, G. P. (1989b). Work, love, and play after brain injury. <u>Bulletin of the Menninger Clinic, 53,</u> 414-431.

Prigatano, G. P. (1992). Personality disturbances associated with traumatic brain injury. <u>Journal of Consulting and Clinical Psychology, 60,</u> 360-368.

Prigatano, G. P. & Klonoff, P. S. (1988). Psychotherapy and neuropsychological assessment after brain injury. <u>Journal of Head Trauma Rehabilitation,</u> <u>3</u>(1), 45-56.

Prigatano, G. P. & Redner, J. E. (1993, February). Uses and abuses of neuropsychological testing in behavioral neurology. <u>Behavioral</u> <u>Neurology, 11</u>(1), 219-231.

*Prigatano, G. P. & Schacter, D. L. (Eds.). (1991). <u>Awareness of deficit after</u> <u>brain injury: Theoretical and clinical issues</u>. New York: Oxford University Press.

Prigatano, G. P., Parsons, O. A. & Bortz, J. J. (1985). Methodological considerations in clinical neuropsychological research: 17 years later. <u>Psychological Assessment, 7</u>(3), 396-403.

*Prigatano, G. P., Klonoff, P. S., O'Brien, K. P., Altman, I. M., Amin, K., Chiapello, D., Shepherd, J., Cunningham, M. & Mora, M. (1994). Productivity after neuropsychologically oriented milieu rehabilitation. <u>Journal of Head Trauma Rehabilitation, 9</u>(1), 91-102.

Prochaska, J. (1991). Assessing how people change. <u>Cancer, 67,</u> 805-807.

*Prochaska, J. & DiClemente, C.C. (1983). Stages and processes of self-change in smoking: Towards an integrative model of change. <u>Journal of</u> <u>Consulting Clinical Psychology, 51,</u> 390-395.

*Prochaska, J. & DiClemente, C.C. (1984). Self change processes, self-efficacy, and decisional balance across five stages of smoking cessation. In P.F. Anderson, L. E. Mortenson & L.E. Epstein (Eds.), <u>Advances in cancer</u> <u>control</u>. New York: Alan R. Liss, Inc.

Prochaska, J. & DiClemente, C.C. (1986). Toward a comprehensive model of change. In W. Miller & N. Heather (Eds.), <u>Treating addictive behaviors</u>. New York,: Plenum Press.

Prochaska, J. & Prochaska, J. M. (1993). A transtheoretical model of change for addictive behaviors. In M. Gossop & M. Casas (Eds.), <u>Recaidaz y</u> <u>Prevencion de Recaidor</u> (pp. 85-136). Sitges, Spain: Citran.

Prochaska, J. O. (1979). <u>Systems of psychotherapy: A transtheoretical analysis</u>. Homeward, IL: Dorsey Press.

*Prochaska, J. O. (1994). Strong and weak principles for progressing from precontemplation to action based on twelve problem behaviors. Health Psychology, 13, 47-51.

*Prochaska, J. O. & DiClemente, C.C. (1985). Common processes of change for smoking, weight control and psychological distress. In S. Shiffman & T. Wills (Eds.), Coping and substance abuse. New York: Academic Press.

Prochaska, J. O. & DiClemente, C.C. (1992). Stages of change in the modification of problem behaviors. In M. Hersen, R. Eisler & P. Miller (Eds.), Progress in Behavior Modification. Sycamore, IL: Sycamore Publishing Co.

*Prochaska, J. O. & Prochaska, J. M. (1995). Why don't continents move?. In H. Arkowitz (Ed.), Why don't people change? New perspectives on resistance and non-compliance. New York: Guilford Press.

*Prochaska, J. O., Rossi, J. S. & Wilcox, N. S. (1991). Change processes and psychotherapy outcome in integrative case research. Journal of Psychotherapy Integration, 1, 103-120.

Prochaska, J. O., DiClemente, C.C. & Norcross, J. (1992). In search of how people change: Application to the addictive behaviors. American Psychologist, 47, 1102-1114.

*Prochaska, J. O., Velicer, W. F., DiClemente, C.C., & Fava, J. (1988). Measuring the process of change: Applications to the cessation of smoking. Journal of Consulting Clinical Psychology, 56, 520-528.

*Prochaska, J. O., DiClemente, C.C., Velicer, W. F., Rossi, J. S. (1993). Standardized, individualized, interactive, and personalized self-help programs for smoking cessation. Health Psychology, 12, 399-405.

*Prochaska, J. O., DiClemente, C.C., Velicer, W. F., Ginpil, S. & Norcross, J. C. (1985). Predicting change in smoking status for self-changers. Addictive Behavior, 10, 395-406.

*Prochaska, J. O., Norcross, J. C., Fowler, J. L., Follick, M. J. & Abrams, D. B. (1992). Attendance and outcome in a work site weight control program: Processes and stages of change as process and predictor variables. Addictive Behavior, 17, 35-45.

*Prochaska, J. O., Redding, C.A., Harlow, L. L., Rossi, J. & Velicer, W. F. (1994, Winter). The transtheoretical model of change and HIV prevention: A review. Health Education Quarterly, 21(4), 471-486.

Prochaska, J. O., Velicer, W. F., Rossi, J. S., Goldstein, M. G., Marcus, B. H., Rakowski, W., Fiore, C., Harlow, L., Redding, C., Rosenbloom, D. & Rossi, S. R. (1994). Stages of change and decisional balance for twelve problem behaviors. Health Psychology, 13, 39-46.

*Rankin, S. H. & Stallings, K. D. (1996). Patient education: Issues, principles, practices. (3rd ed.). Philadelphia: Lippincott.

*Rape, R. N., Bush, J. P. & Slavin, L. A. (1992). Toward a conceptualization of the family's adaptation to a member's head injury: A critique of developmental stage models. Rehabilitation Psychology, 1(37), 3-22.

*Redman, B. K. (1993). The process of patient education (7th ed.). St. Louis: Mosby Year Book.

*Reed, E. S. (1994) Perception is to self as memory is to selves. In U. Neisser & R. Fivush (Eds.), The remembering self: Construction and accuracy in the self-narrative (pp. 278-292). Cambridge: Cambridge University Press.

*Reeve, J. (1996). Motivating others: Nurturing inner motivational resources. Needham Heights, MA: Allyn & Bacon.

*Resnick, L. B. (1991). Shared cognition: Thinking as social practice. In L. B. Resnick, J. M. Levine, & S. D. Teasley (Eds.), Perspectives on socially shared cognition (pp. 1-20). Washington, DC: American Psychological Association.

*Rosenthal, M. & Bond, M. R. (1990). Behavioral and psychiatric sequalae. In M. Rosenthal, E. R. Griffith, M. R. Bond & J. D. Miller (Eds.), Rehabilitation of the adult and child with traumatic brain injury (2nd ed., pp. 179-192). New York: Guilford Press.

*Ross, F. (1991). Patient compliance - Whose responsibility?. Social Science in Medicine, 32(1), 89-94.

*Roth, H. (1987). Current perspectives ten year update on patient compliance research. Patient Education and Counseling, 10, 107-116.

Rubin, S. E. & Rubin, N. M. (Eds.). (1988). <u>Contemporary challenges to the rehabilitation counseling profession</u>. Baltimore: Paul H Brookes Publishing Co., Inc.

*Russell, W. R. (1971). <u>The traumatic amnesias</u>. London: Oxford University Press.

Ryan, M. (1997, July 6). She helps others to fight their way back. <u>Parade Magazine,</u> 10.

*Sachs, P. R. & Redd, C. A. (1993). The Americans with Disabilities Act and individuals with neurological impairments. <u>Rehabilitation Psychology, 38,</u> 87-101.

Saunders, P. (1995, March 1). Encouraging patients to take part in their own care. <u>Nursing Times, 91</u>(9), 42-43.

*Schacter, D. L. & Crovitz, H. F. (1977). Memory function after closed head injury: A review of the quantitative research. <u>Cortex, 13,</u> 150-176.

*Schallert, D. L. (1991). The contribution of psychology to teaching the language arts. In J. Flood, J. M. Jensen, D. Lapp & J. R. Squire (Eds.). <u>Handbook of research on teaching the English language arts</u> (pp. 30-39). New York: Macmillan.

*Schallert, D. L. & Reed, J. H. (1997). The pull of the text and the process of involvement in one's reading. In Guthrie, J. T. & Wigfield, A. (Eds.), <u>Promoting literacy engagement: Motivational, strategic reading through integrated instruction</u> (pp. 68-85). Newark, DL: International Reading Association

Schallert, D. L., Turner, J. E. & McCann, E. J. (1997, March). <u>Engagement in long-term academic tasks: The fluctuating, complementary role of involvement and volition</u>. Paper presented at the annual meeting of the American Educational Research Association, Chicago, IL.

*Schunk, D. H. (1989). Self-efficacy and cognitive skill learning. In C. Ames & R. Ames (Eds.), <u>Research on motivation in education</u> (3) 13-44. San Diego: Academic Press.

Scott, R. (1969). <u>The making of blind men</u>. New York: Russel Sage.

*Seaton, D. (1997, Fall). Editorial. <u>Viewpoints: Issues in Brain Injury Rehabilitation, 36,</u> 1.

*Seaton, S. L., M.D. (Ed.). (1997). <u>Training manual for certified brain injury specialists</u>. Washington, DC: Brain Injury Association.

*Senelick, R. C. & Ryan, C. E. (1991). <u>Living with head injury: A guide for families</u>. Washington, DC: Rehab Hospital Services Corporation.

Sergent, J. (1982). The cerebral balance of power: Confrontation or cooperation. <u>The Journal of Experimental Psychology: Human Perception and Performance, 8,</u> 253-272.

Shotter, J. (1993). A rhetorical-responsive version of social constructionism, Part 1. <u>Conversational realities: Constructing life through language</u>. London: SAGE Publications.

Siegler, M. (1985). The progression of medicine: From physician paternalism to patient autonomy to bureaucratic parsimony. <u>Archives of Internal Medicine, 145,</u> 713-715.

*Shigaki, I. S. (1987). Language and the transmission of values: Implications from Japanese day care. In B. Fillion, C. N. Hedley, & E. C. DiMartino (Eds.), <u>Home and school: Early language and reading,</u> (pp. 111-121). Norwood, NJ: Ablex.

*Shotter, J. (1993). A rhetorical-responsive version of social constructionism, Part 1. In <u>Conversational realities: Constructing life through language</u>. London: SAGE Publications.

*Simkins, C. N. (1994). A relationship between mild to moderate traumatic brain injury and emotional and psychiatric problems. <u>Texas Trial Lawyers Forum, 28</u>(1), 19-21.

*Simon, H. A. (1967). Motivational and emotional controls of cognition. <u>Psychological Review, 74</u>(1), 29-39.

*Simonds, S. (1979). <u>Patient education: A handbook for teachers - National Task Force on Training Family Physicians in Patient Education</u>. Kansas City, MO: The Society for Teachers of Family Medicine.

*Skinner, C. S., Siegfried, J. C., Kegler, M. C., Stretcher, V. J. (1993). The potential of computers in patient education. <u>Patient Education and Counseling, 22,</u> 27-34.

Slife, B. D. & Williams, R. N. (1995). What's behind the research?: Discovering hidden assumptions in the behavioral sciences. Thousand Oaks, CA: SAGE Publications, Inc.

*Slifer, K. J., Babbitt, R. L., Cataldo, M D, Kane, A. C., Harrison, K. A. & Cataldo, M. F. (1993). Behavior analysis and intervention during hospitalization for brain trauma rehabilitation. Archives of Physical Medicine and Rehabilitation, 74, 810-817.

*Smith, N. A., Ley, P., Seale, J. P. & Shaw, J. (1987). Health beliefs, satisfaction and compliance. Patient Education and Counseling, 10, 279-286.

Smith-Knapp, K., Corrigan, J. D. & Arnett, J. A. (1996). Predicting functional independence from neuropsychological tests following traumatic brain injury. Brain Injury, 10(9), 651-661.

Sorrentino, R. M. & Higgins, E. (Eds.). (1986). Handbook of motivation and cognition: Foundations of social behavior. New York: The Guilford Press.

*Spilker, B. (1991). Methods of assessing and improving patient compliance in clinical trials. In J. A. Cramer & B. Spilker (Eds.), Patient compliance in medical practice and clinical trials (pp. 37-56). New York: Raven Press, Ltd.

*Stake, R. E. (1995). The art of case study research. Thousand Oaks, CA: SAGE Publications, Inc.

Steckler, A., Allegrante, J. P., Altman, D., Brown, R., Burdine, J. N., Goodman, R. M. & Jorgensen, C. (1995, August). Health education intervention strategies: Recommendations for future research. Health Education Quarterly, 22(3), 307-328.

Steckler, A., McLeroy, K. R., Goodman, R., Bird, S. T. & McCormick, L. (1992, Spring). Toward integrating qualitative and quantitative methods: An introduction. Health Education Quarterly, 19(1), 1-8.

*Steinmann, Jr., M. (1982). Speech-act theory and writing. What writers know: The language, process, and structure of written discourse (pp. 291-323). New York: Academic Press.

*Stern, B. H. (1996). Opening statement in the mild traumatic brain injury case. Trial Diplomacy Journal, 19, 37-42.

Stipek, D. (1998). <u>Motivation to learn: From theory to practice</u> (3rd ed.). Boston: Allyn and Bacon.

Stratton, M. C. & Gregory, R. J. (1994). After traumatic brain injury: A discussion of consequences. <u>Brain Injury, 8</u>(7), 631-645.

*Strauss, A. & Corbin, J. (1990). <u>Basics of qualitative research: Grounded theory procedures and techniques</u>. Newbury Park, CA: SAGE Publications.

Strecher, V. J., DeVellis, B. M., Becker, M. H. & Rosenstock, I. M. (1986, Spring). The role of self-efficacy in achieving health behavior change. <u>Health Education Quarterly, 13</u>(1), 73-92.

Stuss, D. T. & Buckle, L. (1992). Traumatic brain injury: Neuropsychological deficits and evaluation at different stages of recovery and in different pathologic subtypes. <u>Journal of Head Trauma Rehabilitation, 7</u>(2), 40-49.

Szasz, T.S. & Hollender, M. (1956). The basic models of the doctor-patient relationship. <u>Archives of Internal Medicine, 97,</u> 585-592.

Szymanski, E. M., Buckley, J., Parent, W. S., Parker, R. M. & Westbrook, J. D. (1988). Rehabilitation counseling in supported employment: A conceptual model for service delivery and personnel preparation. In S. E. Rubin & N. M. Rubin (Eds.), <u>Contemporary challenges to the rehabilitation counseling profession</u> (pp. 111-133). Baltimore, MD: Paul H Brooks.

Taylor, S. (1988). Caught in the continuum: A critical analysis of the principle of the least restrictive environment. <u>Journal of the Association for Persons with Severe Handicaps, 13</u>(1), 41-53.

Tickle-Degnen, L. & Rosenthal, R. (1992). Nonverbal aspects of therapeutic rapport. In R. S. Feldman (Ed.), <u>Applications of nonverbal behavioral theories and research</u> (pp. 143-164). Hillsdale, NJ: Lawrence Erlbaum Associates, Publishers.

*Trostle, J. A. (1988). Medical compliance as an ideology. <u>Social Science and Medicine, 27</u>(12), 1299-1308.

Uomoto, J. M. & McLean, A., Jr. (1989). Care continuum in traumatic brain injury rehabilitation. <u>Rehabilitation Psychology, 34</u>(2), 71-79.

*Valenstein, E. & Heilman, K. (1979). Emotional disorders resulting from lesions of the central nervous system. In K. Heilman & E. Valenstein (Eds.), Clinical Neuropsychology). New York: Oxford University Press.

Van Kamerik, S. B. (1978). Why don't patients do what you tell them? Legal Aspects of Medical Practice, 6, 30.

*Vanderhaeghen, C. E. (1985). Self-concept and brain damage. The Journal of General Psychology, 113(2), 139-145.

Vanier, M. (1996). Recovery of speed of information processing in closed-head-injury patients. Journal of Clinical and Experimental Neuropsychology, 18(3), 383-393.

Varney, N. & Menefee, L. (1993). Psychosocial and executive deficits following closed head injury: Implications for orbital frontal cortex. Journal of Head Trauma Rehabilitation, 8(1), 32-44.

*Vendler, Z. (1984). Understanding people. In R. A. Shweder & R. A. LeVine (Eds.), Culture theory: Essays on mind, self, and emotion (pp. 200-213). Cambridge, NY: Cambridge University Press.

*Vygotsky, L. S. (1978). Mind and society: The development of higher mental processes. Cambridge, MA: Harvard University Press.

*Vygotsky, L. (1994). Thought and language. A. Kozulin (Ed.). Cambridge, MA: The MIT Press.

Wehman, P., Kreutzer, J., Wood, W., Morton, M. V. & Sherron, P. (1988). Suppoprted work model for persons with traumatic brain injury: Toward job placement and retention. Rehabilitation Counseling Bulletin, 31, 298-311.

*Weiner, B. (1994). Ability versus effort revisited: The moral determinants of achievement evaluation and achievement as a moral system. Journal Educational Psychologist, 29(3), 163-172.

Weinstein, E. A. & Kahn, R. L. (1955). Denial of illness. Springfield, IL: Charles C. Thomas.

*Wells, G. (1987). The negotiation of meaning: Talking and learning at home and at school. In B. Fillion, C. N. Hedley, & E. C. DiMartino (Eds.), Home and school: Early language and reading (pp. 3-25). Norwood, NJ: Ablex.

*Wertsch, J. V. & Rupert, L. J. (1993). The authority of cultural tools in a sociocultural approach to mediated agency. Cognition & Instruction, 11, 227-239.

Wicker, F. W. & Schallert, D. L. (1996). Involvement as a temporal dynamic: Affective factors in studying for exams. Journal of Educational Psychology, 88, 101-109.

*Willer, B. S., Allen, K. M., Liss, M. & Zicht, M. S. (1991, June). Problems and coping strategies of individuals with traumatic brain injury and their spouses. Archives of Physical Medicine and Rehabilitation, 72, 460-464.

Wolcott, H. F. (1994). Transforming qualitative data: Description, analysis, and interpretation. Thousand Oaks, CA: SAGE Publications.

Woldum, K. M., Ryan-Morrell, V., Towson, M. C., Bower, K. A. & Zander, K. (1985). Patient education: Foundations of practice. Rockville, MD: Aspen Publication.

Wood, R. L. (1987). Brain injury rehabilitation. Rockville, MD: Aspen Publishers, Inc.

*Wuest, J. (1993, September/October). Removing the shackles: A feminist critique of noncompliance. Nursing Outlook, 41, 217-224.

*Yerxa, E. J. (1967). Eleanor Clarke Slagle Lecture: Authentic occupational therapy. American Journal of Occupational Therapy, 21, 1-9.

*Ylvisaker, M. I. & Gobble, E. M. R. (1987). Community reentry for head injured adults. Boston: Little, Brown, and Company Inc.

*Zitney, G. (1995). President's message. TBI Challenge, 3(3/4), 2-3.

Zuger, R. R. & Boehm, M. (1993). Vocational rehabilitation counseling of traumatic brain injury: Factors contributing to stress. Journal of Rehabilition, 59(2), 28-30.

*Zwaagstra, R., Schmidt, I. & Vanier, M. (1996). Recovery of speed of information processing in closed-head-injury patients. Journal of Clinical and Experimental Neuropsychology, 18(3), 383-393.

Vita

Lynda Gail Cleveland was born in Austin, Texas on October 26, 1946, the daughter of Frances Bates Cleveland and Ray O. Cleveland. She obtained her Bachelor of Arts in Speech, English and Drama from Baylor University in Waco, Texas in 1968. She taught at Lake Highlands High School (Richardson ISD), Dallas, following graduation until she entered Texas Tech University in Lubbock, Texas, in 1971 to pursue a Master of Arts degree. Oral interpretation, rhetoric and interpersonal and mass communications were her areas of emphasis for that degree earned in 1973. Returning to Dallas, she taught at Highland Park High School for four years before entering private business. Her business pursuits in the field of audio-visual production and motivational speaking were recognized nationally and internationally.

Lynda is the recipient of numerous state, national and international awards for her excellence in teaching and her skills as a speaker. In addition to her professional lecture appearances, she has shared the motivational dais with speakers such as Paul Harvey, the late Dr. Norman Vincent Peale, Art Linkletter, and Zig Ziglar. Her professional career was cut short in 1984 in a near fatal motor vehicle accident in Melbourne, Australia.

Lynda herself is a survivor of traumatic brain injury and has shared some of her motivational secrets for recovery in her book, *Detour Ahead*. Her concentrated rehabilitation efforts spanned a period of 10 years after which she entered the Graduate School of Biomedical Sciences at The University of Texas Southwestern Medical Center at Dallas in pursuit of a degree in Biomedical

Communications. Following a year of study in Dallas, she continued her doctoral pursuit at The University of Texas at Austin.

Permanent address: 903A The High Road, Austin, Texas 78746

This dissertation was typed by the author with the assistance of Jessye, and was formatted by Pattie F. Rose.

Printed in the United States
107312LV00002B/17/A

9 780977 779598